Nursing Theory

Analysis, Application, Evaluation

• • • •

Fourth Edition

Nursing Theory

Analysis, Application, Evaluation

• • • •

Barbara J. Stevens Barnum, R.N., Ph.D., F.A.A.N.

Editor/Consultant, Nursing Division
Columbia Presbyterian Medical Center
New York, New York

J. B. LIPPINCOTT COMPANY
Philadelphia

Sponsoring Editor: Margaret L. Belcher
Project Editor: Mary Kinsella
Indexer: Ellen Murray
Design Coordinator: Doug Smock
Cover Designer: Anne Bullen
Production Manager: Helen Ewan
Production Coordinator: Maura C. Murphy
Compositor: Bi-Comp, Incorporated
Printer/Binder: R.R. Donnelley & Sons, Crawfordsville
Cover Printer: Leheigh Press

Fourth Edition

6 5 4 3 2 1

Library of Congress Cataloging in Publications Data

Barnum, Barbara Stevens.
    Nursing theory : analysis, application, evaluation / Barbara J.
Stevens Barnum. — 4th ed.
        p.   cm.
    Includes bibliographical references and indexes.
    ISBN 0-397-54942-3
    1. Nursing—Philosophy.   I. Title.
    [DNLM: 1. Nursing Theory.   WY 100 B263n 1994]
    RT84.5.B37   1994
    610.73′01—dc20
    DNLM/DLC
    for Library of Congress   93-12137
                                                                       CIP

Any procedure or practice described in this book should be applied by the
healthcare practitioner under appropriate supervision in accordance with
professional standards of care used with regard to the unique circumstances that
apply in each practice situation. Care has been taken to confirm the accuracy of
information presented and to describe generally accepted practices. However, the
authors, editors, and publisher cannot accept any responsibility for errors or
omissions or for any consequences from application of the information in this book
and make no warranty express or implied, with respect to the contents of the book.

For my mother, Freda Burkett Kushner

Preface to the Fourth Edition

Nursing theory has changed in many ways since the first edition of this book. No longer a strange concept, nursing theory is now discussed in hundreds of books and journals. Extant theories are no longer limited in number but have proliferated on all levels—grand, middle range, and narrow range. Unlike many disciplines, the profession of nursing seems satisfied with a proliferation of conceptual frameworks, though various approaches wax and wane in popularity.

For the student of theory, *Nursing Theory: Analysis, Application, Evaluation, Fourth Edition* provides the tools for understanding, analyzing, and evaluating nursing theories. While most of the popular theories are illustrated and discussed, the book is not intended to serve as a comprehensive survey of theories. Instead, the book should be used along with original works on theory. The reader is strongly encouraged to read original theory formulations rather than secondary interpretations of them, which may or may not be accurate. This book, then, is a work of metatheory—about theory—not a nursing theory itself. *The only intent is to prepare the user to read theory with comprehension.*

This edition, like the previous editions, takes primarily an analytic viewpoint, that is, looking at what has been written about nursing theory and subjecting the writing to semantic analysis. One cannot effectively analyze a theorist—she is a moving target—but one can analyze a given piece of writing.

In this text numerous theory works have been drawn upon to illustrate points of analysis. The reader should not expect that the examples necessarily represent the most recent work of a theorist. Instead, they are works that best illustrate a point being made.

In addition to looking at theory writings, nursing practices that have theoretical implications will be examined. Between analyzing what is written and what is done, it is hoped that the reader will come away effective in applying theory-colored glasses to all endeavors of nursing.

Because readers and the vast majority of theorists in nursing are women, the feminine gender has been used throughout this book. The men of our profession are asked once more to show their flexibility and to accept this choice rather than have every reader face the distortions of content and syntax that result from using the nongendered plural. Theory analysis requires a precision that is often lost when things are stated in the plural.

Finally, the reader will find that the term *theory* is used here to stand for all constructs—paradigms, if you prefer—however complete or tentative in their formulation. People who hold to rigid definitions of what comprises a theory may be uncomfortable with this usage, preferring to reserve the term *theory* for the highest level formulations. Since few theories of nursing have yet reached that pinnacle, I prefer to use the term more liberally, making the point that theory work is important at every level of endeavor.

Barbara J. Stevens Barnum, RN, PhD, FAAN

Contents

Nursing Theory

Analysis, Application, Evaluation

● ● ● ●

1   *What Is Nursing Theory?*

WHAT IS A THEORY?

A *theory* is a construct that accounts for or organizes some phenomenon. A nursing theory, then, describes or explains nursing. It is a shorthand way to characterize a phenomenon, to point out those components or characteristics that give the phenomenon its identity. Theory pulls out the salient parts, separating the critical and necessary factors (or relationships) from the accidental and unessential factors.

A theory is like a map of a territory as opposed to an aerial photograph. The map does not display the full terrain (buildings, moving vehicles, or grazing livestock); instead, it picks out those parts that are important for its purpose. If its aim is to guide travelers, the map will highlight roads; if its purpose is to describe the physical terrain, it shows mountains, plains, and rivers. But no map (or theory) reflects all that is contained within a phenomenon. Such a map would defeat its purpose: giving one a handle on the phenomenon. The handle is created by making the essential parts stand out in relief.

Visintainer (1986) used the map analogy in the following explanation:

> The maps of a discipline operate in a way similar to that of maps of a geographic region. They provide a framework for selecting and organizing information from the environment. In studying a discipline, one learns the maps and through mastery of the maps learns what to ask about, what to observe, what to focus on, what to think about (p. 33).

Different theories of nursing use different maps; that is, diverse components and relationships assume importance in disparate theories. As Visintainer has noted, "Viewing the world through different

Barbara J. Stevens Barnum: NURSING THEORY:
ANALYSIS, APPLICATION, EVALUATION, FOURTH EDITION.
© 1994, 1990, 1984, 1979 J.B. Lippincott.

maps can produce strange twists to a territory with which we are familiar." (p. 35)

There are at least two different types of theories. Some constructs assert something about the way in which its subject exists; others simply give one way in which the thing may be organized. Take, for example, the big bang theory of the universe. This theory proposes something about the creation and subsequent behavior of the universe. It has the potential for being proved or disproved. Similarly, when Einstein's conception of physics replaced Newtonian physics, the new theory corrected errors of fact in the older schema.

Theories of nursing are not constructs of this dimension. Instead, they offer alternate ways in which to describe and organize the content of the discipline. One cannot, for example, say that use of the nursing process and nursing diagnoses (a popular modern theory) is *true*, whereas Orem's self-care theory is *false*. Instead, they represent alternate ways to categorize and make sense of nursing phenomena; they are preferences for organizing thought and action, not irrevocable statements about reality.

TYPES OF THEORY

Theories are classified in many different ways, including their level of development. One such classification simply divides them into those that describe and those that explain.

Descriptive Theory

The *descriptive theory* looks at a phenomenon and identifies its major elements or events (relationships among elements). The theory does not, however, say why the phenomenon has those elements or events, how they relate to each other, or how changes in the elements or relationships affect each other.

In its simplest form, this theory looks at a phenomenon and names its major constituents (elements or events). This lowest level of description is called *ad hoc theory*. Ad hoc theory looks at the phenomenon—for example, let us make it a basket for simplicity—and sees that it contains apples, oranges, and baseballs. It does not explain why baseballs are present with apples and oranges; it merely states that such is the case. The ad hoc theory is primitive, simply pointing out what exists.

When the constituents of a descriptive theory share some structural interrelationship, the theory is termed *categorical* or *classificatory* rather than ad hoc. This is the first effort at sorting what is contained in the theory. Sometimes the relationship among identified elements is one of invariant logical sequence. The nursing process, for example, uses the principle of logical sequence. Patient assessment must precede and lead to diagnosis; diagnosis then leads to the next step, and so forth until the process is completed.

The relationship among theory parts in a categorical descriptive theory usually is one in which the constituents are mutually exclusive and sometimes exhaustive parts. For example, one nursing theory divides the human into separate spiritual, physical, and psychological components.

The theories of King and Levine illustrate the difference between ad hoc and categorical descriptions. King (1981, pp. 10–12) builds a conceptual framework with nursing interacting systems based on personal systems, interpersonal systems, and social systems. Because these systems are based on ever-expanding numbers of interactions (individuals, groups, society), this part of the theory can be labeled as categorical. Yet subcomponents under these labels lack this sort of tidy organization. For example, in relation to personal systems, King has said, "Selected concepts are . . . (1) perception, (2) self, (3) body image, (4) growth and development, (5) time, and (6) space." (p. 10) Obviously these elements are not all one of a kind, so at this level, the theory is ad hoc.

Levine (1971) has used a categorical schema:

> There are four major areas of care in which nursing can fulfill a conservation function. They are embodied in the conservation principles of nursing:
>
> 1. Nursing intervention is based on the conservation of the individual patient's energy.
> 2. Nursing intervention is based on the conservation of the individual patient's structural integrity.
> 3. Nursing intervention is based on the conservation of the individual patient's personal integrity.
> 4. Nursing intervention is based on the conservation of the individual patient's social integrity (p. 258).

Clearly, Levine's four conservation principles (energy, structural integrity, personal integrity, social integrity) are mutually exclusive, but it would be more difficult to assert that they are mutually exhaustive components. Someone might come along and think of a fifth component to be added to the model. Notice Levine's symmetry: all four principles are types of conservation.

The descriptive theory represents the *first level* of work in theory development, that is, it identifies the salient constituents of a theory, naming the elements or events. A descriptive theory may point out complex and abstract concepts, but it is not explanatory if it fails to explain why the phenomenon is as it is or acts as it does. A descriptive theory is an existential statement; it asserts *what is*.

Descriptive theory is not only the first level of theory development but the most important, because it determines what will be perceived as the essence of the phenomenon under study. Subsequent development of a theory will expand on or refine those elements and relationships selected as salient in the descriptive phase. The course of subsequent theory development is channeled by the initial selection of elements seen as critical.

Because most subsequent work on a theory will go into explaining the described elements or events (even if additional elements are added along the way), it is critical that the most significant constituents be recognized and named. Elements and events are not self-evident, so naming is not merely reiteration of the obvious. Even in our example of the basket of apples, oranges, and baseballs, it would have been possible to characterize the phenomenon in different ways, for example, as a collection of red, orange, and white spheres. Given this characterization of the elements, a basket of red jack balls, tangerines, and table tennis balls would be recognized as another instance of the same phenomenon. Yet another description of the basket's contents might characterize them according to size, number, and weight of the elements.

As an exercise in deriving descriptive theory, the reader is invited to see how many different ways our hypothetical basket could be characterized. A few minutes of creative practice will help anyone understand why we have so many radically different constructs by which to describe nursing—a phenomenon far more complex than our basket.

Note that none of these diverse characterizations of the basket needs to be inaccurate. Indeed, the question is not one of right or wrong, but of saliency and significance. What is the most useful way to describe the phenomenon? What parts, in what perspective?

In examining a given descriptive theory, one may ask many important questions such as, Was the perception reflective of reality? In other words, did the theorist see clearly, accurately? Then, what constituents did the author accent? What became foreground, what background? And, did she select the most important constituents? Did she characterize them in the most salient way?

Criteria for determining whether the author succeeded in selecting and characterizing the most important constituents will be discussed later in this book. For now, it will suffice to look briefly at only one criterion: utility. The test of success for a given theory in an applied discipline such as nursing is a practical one. A theory is successful (has selected important constituents) if it is efficient and effective in attaining its socially prescribed goals. In the case of nursing, those goals are outcomes of patient health and comfort that are fully or partly attributable to nursing care. A theory that facilitates the achievement of these nursing goals is successful by the criterion of social utility.

Explanatory Theory

Explanatory theory is the next level in theory development. It attempts to tell how the given constituents of a theory relate to or why they relate with each other. Explanatory theory may deal with cause and effect, correlations, or with the rules that regulate interactions among a theory's constituents. The rules are recognized from study of the patterns established among constituents.

An explanatory theory in its simplest form might assert the following: When Element A interacts with Element B in Manner Q, then Event M inevitably occurs; when Element A interacts with Element B in Manner R, then Event N inevitably occurs. In this case, the rules identify invariant sequences over time. For some subject matter, theories may deal with probabilities (e.g., 90% of the cases), rather than with invariant results. In nursing, there is little that holds true in all cases, except in some cases within the realm of the chemical and biologic.

The test of explanatory theory is whether the prediction holds true in future interactions of the constituents. Some authors designate this stage of explanatory theory as *predictive theory*. If, after formulation of the rule, in every new case Event M follows when Element A interacts with Element B in Manner Q, then the theory has predictive power.

When the phenomenon is such that intervention into constituents is possible, then the theory may be used to control outcomes. Suppose, for example, that Event N is to be preferred over Event M. Then occurrence of N may be fostered by preventing Manner Q or by facilitating Manner R.

When such intervention is possible, leading to a desired outcome versus an undesired one, some authors refer to the controlling theory as *situation producing* (Dickoff, James, & Wiedenbach, 1968, p. 420). Notice that, in these cases, the explanatory theory itself has not changed. What is altered is the use to which it is put, namely, the time when the theory is applied (predictive theory) or the control possible over elements that act according to the theory's rules (situation-producing theory).

The structure of the theory is identical, be it explanatory, predictive, or situation producing. What differs is our faith in it (test of time) or our ability to control its application in the practice setting according to a set of goals. Some authors assume these are differences in degrees of complexity. This is not the case. One might, for example, have a very complex explanation for the rotation of the planets around our sun (explanatory and predictive) without being able to intervene in the planetary system's rotations (situation producing).

EFFECTS OF GOAL DOMINANCE ON THEORY

Most disciplines aim to control their subject matter. In this sense, they are goal directed. But there are two distinct approaches to theory development, and they concern *how* one gains control over one's subject matter. The chemist, for example, aims to find out what the chemical universe is really like. He does not worry about how he *wishes* the chemical universe acted; he tries to find out it *does* act. Once he knows how elements react chemically, then he can create conditions to bring about desired chemical reactions.

Similarly, the sociologist studies what makes people act in certain ways. Again, he may wish that people were different, but he seeks to know how they really *are*. Once he knows how people act, he can (if he has the power) create the conditions that bring about desired behaviors and inhibit undesired ones. If, for example, crowded living conditions produce antisocial acts, the enlightened social planner would design buildings for spaciousness. The chemist and the sociologist accept the realities of the worlds of chemistry and human behavior. They take their domains of inquiry as given.

The nurse theorist seldom approaches her domain in this fashion. If a nurse theorist acted like the chemist, she would say, "There's a universe of nursing out there. I'm going to observe it, identify its major elements and events, then find out what rules account for them."

Once the rules that explained the nursing phenomena were found, by following them, she would produce the desired conditions and eliminate the undesired ones. A few nurses advocate this approach to theory building (Quint, 1967; Schlotfeldt, 1971), but they are in the minority. Chapters 3 through 5 offer some illustrations of deriving theory through observation.

Often nurses have an emotional reaction to theory evolved in this manner and say that the theory may describe what some nurses did, but that it does not describe *nursing*. Here is a clue as to how nursing differs from chemistry, sociology, and many other disciplines. The *source* of nursing for many theorists is not the real world of nursing practice; instead, it is a fantasized ideal world of nursing practice as it *would be* if it were done in the best fashion. In this respect, the nurse theorist is unlike the scientist who first seeks to discover the extant state of his subject matter.

This difference in approach is the reason why values creep into almost every discussion of nursing theory. If the source of nursing is in the *ought to be* rather than the *is*, then the values represented in that *ought* are inseparable from nursing. Goals, in turn, are selected on the basis of the given value system. Hence, in nursing, the value system often dictates both the means and the ends to be pursued.

It is important to recognize that, for most theorists, nursing is a mentally constructed world rather than the real world of nursing practice. When actual nursing behaviors fall short of the preconceived mental image, the theorist says that it may have been done by nurses, but it was not nursing.

The difference between theory development in nursing and in sociology, then, lies in the *locus* of the subject matter. The nursing discipline usually is located in a mental construct of *ought to be*, whereas sociology is located in an extant arena of real events and people.

In analyzing any given nursing theory, the reader must first ask, Does this theory describe nursing as it *is* or as it *ought to be* according to the author? Sometimes an *ought to be* theory is wrongly labeled a situation-producing theory because both are goal dominated. But situation-producing theory also could arise from theory based on *what is*. Most nurse theorists today take their locus for nursing as the *ought*, not the *is*.

DEFINITION OF NURSING

Because the locus of nursing for most theorists is a mental construct rather than an extant arena of real events, it is not that surprising that agreement on a universal definition of nursing is beyond our reach. Indeed, there can be as many mental constructs of nursing as there are nurses to imagine and adopt them. When a construct becomes the criterion for what is and what is not nursing, it is foolhardy to search for universal agreement.

However, one can seek a general consensus on a broad statement concerning nursing. The following might serve that purpose: Nursing is an activity or occasion in which some agent or entity uses its power to aid or manipulate some other agent or entity in relation to aspects of the other agent or entity's health status. The terms in this statement are open-ended in that their meanings may change, based on the perceptions of the person reading the sentence. For example, a nursing *activity* in one theory may involve hands-on care of the body; in another theory, it may represent manipulation of human

behavior. When a term merely points to a broad arena without speci-
fying the content of that arena, it is called a *commonplace*. Such
terms function much like labeled desk drawers into which different
theorists place different contents.

In recent years, nursing theorists have attempted to search for
general areas of agreement among nursing theories, often in an effort
to define a universal theory of nursing. In such an attempt, Fawcett
(1984) has identified the components of person, nursing, health, and
environment. Notice that all these terms are commonplaces and their
definitions will vary from one theory to another. For that reason,
even if nurses agreed on these commonplaces, this would *not* be the
start of a universal theory.

Mistaken perceptions of universal agreement also arise in superficial reading of theory works. Take, for example, the following citation from Newman (1982):

> The major components of nursing theory are man, environment, and
> health. As the nurse interacts with man–environment to facilitate
> health, the nursing process occurs (p. 87).

To the casual reader, this statement may sound as if Newman
were agreeing with Fawcett. On the contrary, if one reads further,
one sees that Newman is using these terms (man, environment, and
health) in very special ways, that is, in a Rogerian style (Rogers,
1990). The terms cannot be taken to have generic meanings as one
might assume from reading the cited sentence out of context. The
difference between a commonplace and a theory element is critical:
an element is specific to a given theory, a commonplace is not. The
reader may wish to see how Flaskerud and Halloran (1980) apply
commonplaces to diverse theories.

Words derive their meaning from their function in a given theory
and from their relationships to other components of that theory. If,
for example, two nurse theorists both use the term *adaptation*, it
cannot be assumed that they mean the same thing by it, nor can it
be assumed that placing the idea of adaptation in a third theory
represents a synthesis of the work of these authors. A term cannot
be borrowed from one theory and put into another without changing
its meaning. Context contributes to a term's meaning; change the
context and you have changed the meaning—even if the word remains.

Another common error in theory development is found at the
opposite end of the continuum, that is, groping for certainty by reducing all theory terms to operational definitions. Although the precise
invariant definition of terms is necessary for research, the same tactic

may cause premature closure on thoughts and ideas in theory work. For example, if one operationally defines the term *patient* before developing a nursing theory, the direction in which that theory may go has already been crystallized. In theory development, an initial tolerance for ambiguity is desirable.

More important, terms may lose the richness of their meaning when operationalized for research. Take the term *adolescence*. It might be operationalized by setting an arbitrary age limit or by validating the occurrence of specified physiologic and sociologic boundary events. But these operationalized definitions are not meant to convey the full significance of the term; they are only meant to enable the researcher to differentiate an adolescent from other people. Although essential for research, operationalized terms can limit conceptualization in theory development.

For the purposes of this book, the reader is asked to suspend the learned desire for a concise definition. The reader should recognize that the term *nursing* points only to a general arena of events and that its specific meaning will be different in every nursing theory.

Boundaries

Although it is necessary to tolerate ambiguity in any shared definition of nursing, it is important that any specific nursing theory—directly or implicitly—differentiate nursing from other disciplines and activities. Many so-called theories of nursing fail in this aspect, creating a schema that could apply equally well to medicine, physical therapy, social work, or other endeavors. These theories have failed to settle the boundary issue. When held separate from specific content, the so-called nursing process can be criticized for this fault. The electrical engineer, the architect, the nuclear scientist, as well as the school counselor could claim that they assess, diagnose, plan, intervene, and evaluate. One could easily talk about the architectural process or the counseling process. Only when this common process is tied to specific content (additional theory elements) can one say the boundary has been drawn successfully around a discipline. When authors fail to differentiate nursing, the error usually is found in one of two directions: either the theory is equally applicable to (1) medicine and other health professions or (2) nonprofessional activities such as mothering, caring, and nurturing.

Theories based on stress-adaptation models often err in failing to differentiate nursing from other health professions. When reading a theory work, a good test for this error is to substitute the word *medicine* (or social work) for the word *nursing* every time it appears.

If the work remains cogent and applicable in the substituted discipline, then the theory has failed to distinguish nursing from other health professions.

A theory that defines nursing primarily by its intent or effect, without reference to the skills unique to nursing, may fail in the opposite direction, that is, not differentiating nursing from the general caring acts of humans for one another. Some theories based on caring models fall into this error. Try substituting terms such as *mother* or *caring human* for *nurse* in these theories to test for the flaw.

BASIS FOR BOUNDARIES

When a theory successfully differentiates nursing from other disciplines and human activities, it is important to ask the basis of that differentiation. Is nursing unique because it has a separate body of knowledge? Because it uses shared knowledge in a distinct manner? Because it comes into being in a unique set of circumstances? Or because it has discrete goals?

The first interpretation differentiates nursing in terms of its substantive *content*; the second in terms of its method and practices, that is, *processes*; the third in terms of the *context* in which it occurs; and the last in terms of its *goals*. Each interpretation presents its own difficulties.

Where nursing's uniqueness lies in knowledge (content) rather than in action, defining the unique body of knowledge is tricky. Yet, if the locus of nursing is its content, the knowledge must be separate and unlike that taught in other health disciplines. The problem here is one of finding knowledge so unique that no other discipline lays claim to it. Rogers (1990, p. 6), for example, asserted that nursing's unique subject matter is the science of unitary human beings—man in his totality rather than seen in component parts.

When a nursing theory develops a truly unique body of knowledge, it has another problem—that of communicating its meaning to other health disciplines. When nursing's subject matter is radically different, its distinct language may present interface problems in situations in which different professions work closely together. This does not mean that nursing cannot develop separate theories; it simply means that one considers what is to be gained and what is to be lost in this tactic. In adopting a theory that has a radically different conceptualization of man (or his care) than the theories used by other health workers in the care environment, one runs the danger of increasing problems in interprofessional communication.

When a radically divergent nursing theory is selected, nursing has the task of helping others understand its unique language or of translating its programs into language that others can understand. Where communication bridges are not devised, cooperative work is difficult. Many theorists argue, however, that creating separate content for nursing is worth the price of problematic communications because it establishes a clear and separate identity for nursing.

When nursing's uniqueness lies in the *use* of knowledge rather than in the knowledge per se, another set of problems emerges. One must show how nursing bridges shared content and unique action, and one must identify which acts are particularized to nursing and why. What groups share the content that each applies differently? Medicine? Social work? How is the application different?

Some theories that find nursing's boundaries in its *use* of knowledge see it as a generalist practice arising from the blending of content from other disciplines. Where this interpretation is given, the difficulty is in explaining how one can synthesize content from various disciplines (e.g., medicine, anatomy, psychology, and sociology) when the nurse is not an expert in any of them. Here, the nurse theorist faces the awesome task of explaining how one derives a generalist's discipline from little-studied specialty fields.

Perhaps the most difficult boundary to understand is where the *circumstance* (or context) differentiates nursing from other disciplines. In written theories, a context often is assumed rather than stated. Some theorists, for example, have an underlying image of nursing as constituted by all those acts between nurse and patient in an acute care hospital setting. In this example, an act becomes nursing, not because of its content or method, but because it occurs in a particular setting where a nurse and patient are brought together.

Take a different context: suppose a nurse is talking to a neighbor who asks about a health-related problem. When does *nursing*, as opposed to casual conversation, begin? Or does it? What situational variants define the context as a nursing situation?

Theory is not easier if the difference is to be made on the basis of *goals*. Here, a unique complexity arises because nursing contributes toward achievement of medical as well as nursing goals. When a nurse performs an act aimed toward medical goals, is she nursing? If not, what is she doing? Chinn and Jacobs (1983) differentiate nursing from medicine in the following goal-focused way:

> *The value of inclusions or exclusions of areas of inquiry is determined by assessing how valuable the inquiry is in reaching the goals of the discipline. Thus if a discipline holds the goal of curing disease, those*

human responses to health problems that are related to this goal will be studied. If the concern of the discipline is the human response to problems created by disease, then the phenomena studied will be both similar to and different from a discipline concerned with curing disease (p. 19).

For all theories of nursing, it is important to ask whether the uniqueness is identified, characterized, simply asserted, or put forth as something to be found in future work and research. Where the uniqueness is projected to arise out of future work and research a theory is necessarily incomplete and vague. For any given theory one may ask,

1. How does nursing in this theory differ from other disciplines and actions?
2. What is the basis of nursing's uniqueness?
3. Is that uniqueness identified or merely asserted?

When a theory is well developed, it will explain the content, methods, context, and goals of nursing, whether they be unique or shared. Initially many theories focus on one or two of these aspects to the exclusion of others. The reader may wish to practice identifying these underlying elements (stated or unstated, included or ignored) when reading theory materials. Even nontheory works in nursing are set in the context of an author's conceptualization of nursing and may be analyzed accordingly. In reading theory, unlike most other works, it is just as important to notice what *is not* there as what *is.*

COMPARING THEORIES

When the elements of several theories are sorted into commonplaces, it is possible to compare and contrast them. Content, methods, context, and goals can serve as the bins in our sorting exercise. Keep in mind that a theory may ignore certain common sorting bins while having important concepts requiring the addition of new sorting categories. Because separating a theory's components by content, method, context, and goal may be difficult, some alternate lists of commonplaces are suggested.

For each commonplace in a set, one asks, Given this particular theory, what, if anything, fits into this particular container? The set of containers addressed and omitted, taken together, tells the reader much about the given theory.

Theory analysts create their own sets of commonplaces, and there is no one right set. Analysts concerned with adequacy tend to produce long lists of commonplaces; those concerned with parsimony produce short lists. In their classical work, Dickoff et al. (1968) used the following commonplaces:

Agency: Who or what performs the activity?
Patiency: Who or what is the recipient of the activity?
Framework: In what context is the activity performed?
Terminus: What is the end point of the activity?
Procedure: What is the guiding procedure, technique, or protocol of the activity?
Dynamics: What is the energy source for the activity? (p. 423)

Patiency is a good example from this list. Virtually every nursing theory has some concept of a patient, but the meaning may differ radically from one theory to another. In one, a patient may be a discrete person. Another theory may label a group, community, or organizational entity as patient. Yet another theory may characterize a patient by his entering into a particular type of relationship with a nurse. Another may characterize a patient by specific manifest health needs. One theory may classify the wife of a hospitalized person as *patient* when she learns to balance meals for her diabetic mate. Another theory may claim that patiency resides only in the husband with the health problem.

Duffey and Muhlenkamp (1974) offered a different list of commonplaces—questions that form the basis for their evaluation of nursing theories:

What is the origin of the problems with which the theory is concerned?
What are the methods used?
What is the character of the subject matter dealt with by the theory?
What kind of outcomes of testing propositions generated by this theory would you expect to get? (p. 571)

Roy (1980) consciously used commonplaces in the *construction* of her theory, identifying the following commonplaces:

Values
Goals of action
Patiency of the recipient
Source of difficulty
Intervention (pp. 183–187)

All these commonplaces, as well as Fawcett's, could be used for evaluating theories or as structures for organizing a theory by the author–theorist.

In each case, the selected commonplaces tell something about their creator's perspective on nursing. In this sense, the subjective aspect cannot be totally avoided. In addition to analyzing the contents that fall within a set of commonplaces, the reader can analyze the advantages and limitations inherent in any given set of commonplaces.

The following set of commonplaces are used for theory analysis in this book: nursing acts, the patient, health, the relationship of nursing acts to the patient, the relationship of nursing acts to health, and the relationship of the patient to health. Here, commonplaces are reduced to three elements (nursing acts, the patient, and health) and their interrelationships. With this set, one would ask such questions as,

1. Of what do nursing acts consist in the given theory? What is the nature of nursing? Who is able to perform nursing acts?
2. Who or what is the patient in the given theory?
3. What is meant by health in this theory? What is meant by wellness and illness? What is the image of health held by the author?
4. What is the relationship between nursing acts and the patient? Between nurse and patient?
5. What is the relationship between nursing acts and health? In what way does nursing contribute to health?
6. What is the relationship of the patient to health? How does the patient attain or approach it?

These commonplaces were selected primarily for parsimony. Variations in what the commonplace *patient* means have been illustrated, as have variations in *nursing acts,* for example, cognitive acts, behavioral tasks, hands-on care. *Health* has different meanings, too. For one theorist, it may represent a full continuum of states of being, ranging from illness to wellness. For another, it may be discussed only in the context of ill health, arising only in a state of deficiency or in the presence of a health problem.

NURSING ACT, PATIENT, AND INTERACTION

Theories also differ as to which commonplaces are stressed. Most nursing theories place their basic principles in one of three loci:

1. the nursing act
2. the patient
3. the relationship between patient and nursing act (the interaction itself)

In the first instance, the unstated assumption is that by knowing what the nurse does (or should do) one comes to understand nursing.

The second focus implies that if we really understand the patient, then knowledge of nursing acts logically follows. The third stance does not place the essence of nursing in the acts or conditions of any human agent, but in the particular character of the interchange between patient and nurse.

Major trends in nursing as well as major nursing theories can be attributed to these three alternative emphases. For example, the focus on the nurse and what she does is illustrated by the nursing process. The American Nurses' Association's (ANA's) advocacy of the nursing process (it appears in almost all ANA standards of practice) has done much to make the nursing act dominant.

In contrast, a focus on the patient is evident in nursing curricula structured around body systems. Here, if one knows the patient, namely his body systems, the correct nursing acts logically will follow. Curricula based on patient problems (pain, anxiety, immobility) also select the patient as the focus.

Curricula and practice based on nursing diagnoses often mix these two elements in disorderly array. For example, a nursing diagnosis of respiratory distress is centered in the patient, whereas a diagnosis of negative appraisal by others (Carpenito, 1984, p. 74) may be more the nurse's problem.

A focus on the interaction itself is evident in the works of King and Watson. King's (1981) approach is existential, confirming that interaction occurs between patient and nurse, with *transaction* (agreement between patient and nurse on a goal with movement toward achievement of the goal) as the culminating act (pp. 60–62). Watson's (1988) notion of caring creates a different sort of interaction theory. Her transaction simultaneously contributes to the patient's and the nurse's development of spiritual essence, self-knowledge, and self-healing (p. 57).

INTERPRETING NURSING THEORIES

Theorists do not make the job of identifying commonplaces easy. Seldom will a theorist state, in so many words, that her image of a patient is a hospitalized individual under medical care. Yet, if every reference to patient were given from this perspective, and nursing, as described, occurs only when a person is in this state, then the reader can infer that this description of patient (patiency) fits.

One also cannot take a theorist too literally. For example, she may start out with a definition of patient as an individual, group of people, or community. But if all further discussion only addresses the patient as an individual, then the theorist's original definition was simply a slogan. The real definition is *that characterization intrinsic to the given theory.*

Many theorists fall into the trap of using slogans, particularly those in vogue at the time their material was written. One sees theorists who claim that the patient is a full-fledged participant in determining his plan of nursing care, yet fail to apply the concept in the theory that follows. *Sloganism* is a claim put forth but not substantiated in the theory elaboration. The reader may be suspicious of any of the following six claims until substantiated:

1. the nurse is a problem solver
2. the patient participates in his care determination
3. health is a state of total well-being
4. the nurse uses the nursing process
5. the theory uses a systems approach to nursing
6. caring is the basis of all nursing actions.

SUMMARY

There are many structural devices that enable the reader to understand theory and to compare and contrast theories in a systematic fashion. These devices include, among others, determining whether the theory is descriptive or explanatory—as well as its level of development within that categorization. Further, the reader can determine the boundaries that divide nursing from other activities for any given theory, as well as considering the commonplaces addressed or omitted and the meanings given to each commonplace used.

Other schemas for viewing a theory include identifying its various elements as content, process, or context. Similarly, one can determine whether a theory's principles are based on the nursing act, the patient, or their interaction.

Learning to interpret theory through the devices presented in this chapter takes time, but ultimately the analytic devices will help the reader to grasp the nature of nursing theory. Theory must be understood in all its complexities if it is to be applied in one's work; a theory can't simply be memorized like a procedure. Hence these analytic tools are not presented as a burden but as a means for enhancing one's understanding of the theories that will be discussed in the rest of this book.

PRACTICE EXERCISE

The reader may wish to apply the content of this chapter to an analysis of one or more theories. Pick any theories that interest you, but use works of limited size, perhaps four to six pages. An initial analysis will require several readings. Carefully read and reread the given theory piece, asking the following questions or completing the identified tasks.

1. *Identify the major elements of the theory.*
   Which commonplace elements are present? Which are missing?
2. *Identify relationships among the elements.*
   Are relationships described? Can elements be categorized, classified, sequenced?
3. *Determine whether the theory is descriptive or explanatory.*
   Does the theory simply tell what exists? Does the theory tell why and how?
4. *Determine if the theory describes nursing as it is or as it should be.*
   Does the theory describe what nurses do or what nurses ought to do?
5. *Give a definition of nursing that summarizes the theory.*
   Is the definition stated in the writing? Or can one infer it from the given theory elements?
6. *Tell how nursing in this theory differs from other domains.*
   Does the theory also distinguish nursing from medicine or other health fields? Does it distinguish nursing from other aspects of life unrelated to health per se (e.g., normal social interaction)?
7. *Tell how nursing differs from simple caring acts.*
   Must one be a professional nurse to nurse in the sense implied by the theory? Or could a nurse's aide or a licensed practical nurse perform a nursing act? Could a mother provide nursing according to this theory?
8. *Tell whether the crux of nursing rests in the content of nursing knowledge, in the methods of performing nursing acts, in the nursing context, or in its goals.*
   How many of these elements are addressed or assumed? Which are ignored? Which is most important in characterizing nursing?
9. *For this theory, give the stated or implied meanings of each commonplace:*
   a. Nursing acts
   b. Patient
   c. Health
   d. Relationship between nursing acts and patient
   e. Relationship between nursing acts and health
   f. Relationship between patient and health
   Try a different set of commonplaces if you so choose.

10. *Identify the main locus of the theory: patient, nursing act, or nurse–patient relationship.*
   Do the elements defined in the first task support your conclusion? Do the terms used by the author focus on the patient (or elements of his being); the nurse (or her acts); or the relationship between patient and nurse?
11. *Identify slogans used by the author.*
   Did the theorist give any definitions inconsistent with the theory? Were any claims asserted and then dropped from subsequent discussion?

REFERENCES

Carpenito, L. J. (1984). *Handbook of nursing diagnosis.* Philadelphia: J. B. Lippincott.

Chinn, P. L., & Jacobs, M. K. (1983). *Theory and nursing: A systematic approach.* St. Louis, MO: C.V. Mosby.

Dickoff, J., James, P., & Wiedenbach, E. (1968). Theory in a practice discipline: Part I. Practice oriented theory. *Nursing Research, 5,* 415–435.

Duffey, M., & Muhlenkamp, A. F. (1974). A framework for theory analysis. *Nursing Outlook, 9,* 571–574.

Fawcett, J. (1984). The metaparadigm in nursing: Present status and future refinements. *Image, 3,* 84–87.

Flaskerud, J. H., & Halloran, E. J. (1980). Areas of agreement in nursing theory development. *Advances in Nursing Science, 1,* 1–7.

King, I. M. (1981). *A theory for nursing: Systems, concepts, process.* New York: Wiley.

Levine, M. E. (1971). Holistic nursing. *Nursing Clinics of North America, 2,* 253–264.

Newman, M. A. (1982). What differentiates clinical research? *Image, 3,* 86–88.

Quint, J. C. (1967). The case for theories generated from empirical data. *Nursing Research, 2,* 109–114.

Rogers, M. E. (1990). Nursing: Science of unitary, irreducible, human beings: Update 1990. In E.A.M. Barrett (Ed.), *Visions of Rogers' science-based nursing* (pp. 5–11). New York: National League for Nursing.

Roy, C. (1980). The Roy adaptation model. In J. P. Riehl & C. Roy (Eds.), *Conceptual models for nursing practice* (2nd ed., pp. 179–188). New York: Appleton-Century-Crofts.

Schlotfeldt, R. M. (1971). The significance of empirical research for nursing. *Nursing Research, 2,* 140–142.

Visintainer, M. A. (1986). The nature of knowledge and theory in nursing. *Image, 2,* 32–38.

Watson, J. (1988). *Nursing: Human science and human care: A theory of nursing.* New York: National League for Nursing.

BIBLIOGRAPHY

Bohny, B. J. (1980). Theory development for a nursing science. *Nursing Forum, 1,* 51–67.

Capers, C. F. (1986). Some basic facts about models, nursing conceptualizations, and nursing theories. *Journal of Continuing Education in Nursing, 5,* 149–154.

Chinn, P. L. (1987). Response: Re vision and passion. *Scholarly Inquiry for Nursing Practice, 1,* 21–24.

Hardy, L. K. (1986). Identifying the place of theoretical frameworks in an evolving discipline. *Journal of Advanced Nursing, 1,* 103–107.

Jacobson, S. F. (1987). Studying and using conceptual models of nursing. *Image, 2,* 78–82.

Lancaster, W., & Lancaster, J. (1981). Models and model building in nursing. *Advances in Nursing Science, 3,* 31–42.

Meleis, A. I. (1987). Re visions in knowledge development: A passion for substance. *Scholarly Inquiry for Nursing Practice, 1,* 5–19.

Meleis, A. I. (1991). *Theoretical nursing: Development and progress* (2nd ed.). Philadelphia: J.B. Lippincott.

Walker, L. O., & Avant, K. C. (1988). *Strategies for theory construction in nursing* (2nd ed.). Norwalk, CT: Appleton & Lange.

2 *Structure Underlying Theory*

COMPREHENSIVE THEORY ELEMENTS

Chapter 1 mentioned the use of context, content, and process as tools for analyzing works of nursing theory. This chapter examines these notions in greater detail, providing examples that use these notions to analyze and compare theories.

A complete theory of nursing identifies all three elements: context, content, and process. I like to envision these elements as a carpet on which a design has been embossed. The original unadorned rug may be equated with the context, that is, the background on which the other elements play. The threads of the embossed design are envisioned to crosshatch so that those running horizontally represent content, whereas those running vertically may be equated with process. Content and process interact on the background, that is, the context. A fourth element, goals, is not discussed in this chapter because of its complexity for the theory beginner. But to complete the analogy, goals could be seen to equate with the direction in which the rug itself is faced.

In brief, context is the *environment* in which nursing acts occur. It tells the nature of the world of nursing and, in many cases, describes the nature of the patient or his world. For example, Roy (1980) has stated that she sees a world characterized by the dominance of stimulus–response reactions. In this sort of world, the nurse manipulates stimuli; the patient responds.

Content is the *subject matter* of a theory; it comprises the stable components that are acted on or that do the acting. For example,

Barbara J. Stevens Barnum: NURSING THEORY:
ANALYSIS, APPLICATION, EVALUATION, FOURTH EDITION.
© 1994, 1990, 1984, 1979 J.B. Lippincott.

Levine (1967, 1971) has offered energy, structure, personal integrity, and social integrity as her content components. Process is the *method* by which the nurse acts in using the theory. She acts on, with, or through the content pieces of the theory. See Appendix A, for example, where Hall (1966) offered *mirroring* as a major nursing method; that is, the nurse holds up to the patient a reflection of his own behavior. King's (1981) theory has a process shared by the nurse and patient, resulting in action, reaction, and transaction. Each of these elements—context, content, and process—are addressed in more detail so that the reader can become comfortable with their use.

CONTEXT

What counts as significant *context* differs from theory to theory. It may be the nature of the planet itself (e.g., in ecofeminism); it may be the nature of the patient's immediate environment (e.g., the acute care hospital world); or it may be the nature of humans themselves (as in Roy's stimulus–response connotation). Whatever context is important to a theory, it describes the nature of the background on which nursing occurs.

Johnson (1980) has a context whereby the nurse works in a world of behavior. The patient exhibits behaviors; the nurse manipulates to create desired changes in behavior. This does not mean that the entire universe is made up only of behavior, but for Johnson, behavior is the domain in which nursing occurs. In contrast, Rubin (1968) has a context described as the eternally changing present. The idea of the moment and the fluidity of circumstances characterize the environment for her. For Leininger (1991), the patient's culture is the important context. Some theorists spell out context better than others. Watson (1988) specifically defined the human science context in which her theory is located:

- a philosophy of human freedom, choice, responsibility
- a biology and psychology of holism (nonreducible persons interconnected with others and nature)
- an epistemology that allows not only for empirics, but for advancement of esthetics, ethical values, intuition, and process discovery
- an ontology of time *and* space
- a context of interhuman events, processes, and relationships
- a scientific world view that is open (p. 16).

After one reads such a list, it is easy to imagine the sort of nursing that would fit—or not fit—in such a world.

Context is not always captured in a single notion or a finite set of principles like Watson's. In Hall's theory (see Appendix A), it is accurate to say that her context is chronic illness. It is also accurate to say that her context is one of existential crisis in which man's capacity for radical free choice characterizes the environment. Both of these aspects would be accurate reflections of context.

Chopoorian (1986) noted that there are many significant environments, for example,

1. the social, political, and economic structures
2. human, social relations
3. everyday life (pp. 47–53).

Clearly, a theory of nursing can present many different yet not inconsistent environments. Context is the category that extracts the most important environments, the ones that are essential to understanding the theory. In many nursing theories, the context is unstated and must be inferred from the general discussion. For example, one might find a theory in which the context is the acute care hospital dealing with ill patients. In a better detailed theory, one might find a context of health deficit or one in which homeostasis is the key to the patient's world. These examples, both illness based, might be contrasted with a theory in which even the well need nursing.

Donovan (1970) is one of the rare theorists who has carefully identified context. She classified sources of nursing by contextual factors:

1. derived—through the medical plan
2. fluctuating—relinquished from others (e.g., the pharmacist)
3. coordinative—elements resulting from the holding position of the nurse in relation to the patient
4. independent—those elements that are distinctly nursing (pp. 12–15).

Finer (1952, pp. 88, 90) has given a different description of context in nursing. He noted that nursing occurs in an environment characterized by continuousness, diversity of needs, contingency, and high emotionality. By continuous, he meant the nurse's 24-hour uninterrupted vigilance over the patient. By diversity of needs, he meant the need to individualize patient care planning. Contingency refers to the ever-changing nature of the patient's needs, and the fact that nursing acts must be adjusted on an ongoing basis. High emotionality refers to the life-and-death and stress-filled situations faced by patients, requiring compassion and understanding on the part of the nurse.

More recently Leininger (1991, p. 43), in her ethnonursing model, broke out cultural and social context including structures of technological factors, religious and philosophical factors, kinship and social factors, cultural values and lifeways, political and legal factors, economic factors, and educational factors.

The differences in context among theorists illustrate a shift over time in the nursing viewpoint. Older theories like those of Donovan and Finer tended to have the image of an acute care hospital in mind when creating theory. Newer theories, like Leininger's or Chopoorian's, tend to see nursing in a broader context. In a time when much nursing care is shifting from the acute care setting to home and community, this shift in theory context is to be expected.

CONTENT

The term *content* is used in this chapter to identify the relatively stable theory elements that are the subject matter of a nursing theory. Often the subject elements are the categories through which nursing acts are accomplished. For Johnson (1980), content consists of the categories of patient behavior: elimination behavior, sexual behavior, and so forth. For Roy (1980), content would include the four adaptation modes of man: (1) physiologic needs, (2) self-concept, (3) role function, and (4) interdependence relations. For Neuman (1980), content would include, but would not be limited to, energy resources, stressors, and lines of resistance.

Not all theorists contain their basic content to aspects of the patient. For King (1981), one set of content items would be personal systems, interpersonal relationships, and social systems. Rogers's (1970) components are even broader, consisting of man (human field); environmental field; space; time; and innovation. Content intersects with both process and context to make a complete theory. The interaction with process may be illustrated in the theories built around the so-called nursing process. In this theory (there are many variations on the theme), the nursing process (assess, diagnose, intervene, evaluate) is linked to a taxonomy of nursing diagnoses. These diagnoses, the most common arising from the work of the North American Nursing Diagnosis Association (1989), represent the content part of the theory.

For an excellent example of content interacting with context, see Strauss, Fagerhaugh, and Glaser (1974). These authors, in a narrow range theory, considered the content (pain) as it was affected by context (the "normal" pain trajectories for the given work areas). They found that different areas in the same institution (altered contexts) dealt with pain in radically different ways.

Content items, then, are the main building blocks that give a theory form without being the moving forces. The moving forces constitute the processes.

PROCESS

Processes may be stated as nouns or verbs, but in either case, they represent the movement, the action part of the theory. The processes (or process) of a theory refer to those activities (intellectual, affective, or behavioral) on the part of the agent (nurse or patient) that are required to implement the theory. For Hall (1966), process elements include mirroring, nurturing, and comforting on the part of the nurse and self-mastery on the part of the patient. For Levine (1971), nurses conserve; patients adapt. For Newman (1979), the nurse helps the patient expand his consciousness by "[assisting] people to utilize the power that is within them as they evolve toward higher levels of consciousness." (pp. 66–67)

Almost invariably, the process items of a theory act on or through the content items of the theory. For example, in Orem (1985), self-care (an action; that is, a process) is applied in the content domains of air, water, and food; excrements; rest and activity; and so forth (p. 92). Roy (1980), in contrast, operates on a microlevel. Her nurse manipulates stimulus–response (process) in the content domains of physiologic needs, self-concept needs, role function, and interdependence (p. 182).

For some theorists, process is reduced to a single activity, for example, problem solving. For others, numerous processes are involved. Orem (1985) illustrated both points, because her theory is based on a major process: self-care. Yet the specific forms for self-care differ with each content item. For example, she spoke of maintenance (process) of sufficient intake of air; water; food (content); or provision of care (process) associated with eliminative processes and excrements (content) (p. 92).

In yet another section of her book, Orem (1985) classified those processes in a different manner, according to the method of giving assistance:

1. Acting for or doing for another
2. Guiding another
3. Supporting another (physically or psychologically)
4. Providing an environment for another that promotes personal development in relation to becoming able to meet present or future demands for action
5. Teaching another (p. 138).

Two common process theory threads in nursing are the nursing process and problem solving. Both are discussed in detail in later chapters. For now, it is enough to note that either of these processes may be combined with differing contents and offered in varied contexts. Keep in mind that the processes will be somewhat changed according to the context and content in which they are combined.

Other processes are certainly possible in nursing; they are just not as common. It is surprising, for example, that nursing has not created a popular theory based on the method of differential diagnosis as has been done in medicine. Orem's original theory comes closest to this operational pattern, that is, making either/or choices at each step.

In some theories, the dialectic process of synthesis is the method of choice. The term *synthesis* often is used in nursing literature, but the process itself is not as often used in practice. Sometimes nurses claim to be synthesizing when they are actually accumulating (adding) data or activities.

Brodt (1980) is one theorist who used the notion of synthesis or synergism accurately. However, she used it in relation to goal achievement rather than in relation to a nursing process. She said,

> The synergistic theory of nursing postulates that nursing practice consists of six dimensions of practice, which when delivered to the client simultaneously and interrelatedly provide the optimum level of care and the most positive outcome for the client. . . .
>
> As a corollary, the effect of each dimension of nursing practice enhances the other dimensions when presented simultaneously and interrelatedly. The effect is similar to the synergistic action of two drugs on the human body, in which the combined action is different from the effect of either drug taken independently. In the combined administration of the nursing dimensions, the whole also is greater than the sum of its parts (pp. 85, 87).

The dimensions of Brodt's theory include preservation of body defenses, prevention of complications, maintenance or reestablishment of the client with the outside world, detection of changes in the body's regulatory system, implementation of the physician's prescribed therapy, and provision of comfort and safety. Notice that each item contains both content and process. This format was common in early theory works in which each process was identified with a specific content. Thus, we see that, for Brodt, preservation (process) relates to body defenses (content); prevention (process) relates to complication (content); and so forth. Compare this with the newer format in which one process—for example, conservation—is applied to numerous categorical (not ad hoc) content items.

Although Brodt (1980) has described synthesis as a *result*, Newman (1979) has described it as a dialectic *process:*

> A holistic approach is not to be confused with, or construed to mean, a multivariate approach. It is not the summing up of many factors (psychological, social, physiologic, and so on) to make a whole. It is the identification of patterns which are reflective of the whole (p. 70).

Not surprisingly, Newman claims that phenomenology offers nurses the opportunity to observe these patterns of the whole. As with Newman, the process in a given theory not only tells how the nurse performs (intellectually or behaviorally) as practitioner, but also indicates appropriate methods of research and teaching behavior. For the same theory, processes in these domains should be consonant if not identical.

Often the processes of a theory are termed its *syntactical structures*. As Ziman (1968) has said,

> To understand the nature of Science, we must look at the way in which scientists behave toward one another, how they are organized and how information passes between them. The young scientist does not study formal logic, but he learns by imitation and experience a number of conventions that embody strong social relationships (p. 10).

INTERPLAY

Few theories are complete in their descriptions of context, content, and process. Theorists often focus on one or two of these structural constituents, giving minimal attention to the remaining. Donovan (1970) and Finer (1952) stressed context. Johnson (1980) stressed content (e.g., behavioral systems). On the other hand, her attention to process was less well formulated:

> Nursing is thus seen as an external regulatory force which acts to preserve the organization and integration of the patient's behavior at an optimal level under those conditions in which the behavior constitutes a threat to physical or social health, or in which illness is found. This force operates through the imposition of external regulatory or control mechanisms, through attempts to change structural units in desirable directions, or through the fulfillment of the functional requirements of the subsystems (p. 214).

In contrast to Johnson's brief clarification of how her processes of nursing are applied, Peplau (1989) detailed her process. For example, in a psychiatric nursing context, she spelled out the unique processes for managing frustration, anxiety, and other phenomena.

Given the content of patient anxiety, she identified process steps to accompany every aspect of the patient experience (pp. 24–25). For example, when the patient makes an expectation operative, the nurse connects the anxiety and the expectation (process). When the patient subsequently experiences discomfort and internal tension, the nurse names the experience as anxiety. Peplau continued this step-by-step approach throughout the whole anxiety experience, with nursing process tied to each step of the patient's experience. Notice that we really have two processes at work in Peplau's discussion: the patient's experiential process and the nurse's response process. One of the charms of Peplau for many nurses is that her work gives these concrete steps to be taken. Others, however, are frustrated by the number of components that thereby accrue in her work.

Just as Peplau found processes in both the patient and nurse, so Levine found the reciprocal processes of adaptation (on the part of the patient) and conservation (on the part of the nurse). But the activation principles in Levine's early writing were not so well developed as Peplau's directives. For example, Levine (1967) said,

> The integrated response of the individual to any stimulus results in a realignment of his very substance, and in a sense this creates a message which others may learn to understand. Each message, in turn, is the result of observation, selection of relevant data, and assessment of the priorities demanded by such knowledge (p. 46).

This single statement is the only indication of how the conservation process is structured in the given citation. This format, incidentally, is typical of a problematic method. Seldom do problematic methods spell out methods, because different methods may be used to solve different problems.

In contrast, Levine's later work (1973, pp. 7–9) detailed the patient's process (maintaining a homeostatic balance between an upper and lower normal limit) and the nurse's intervention (exercising control over negative feedback in regulatory systems). In this later citation, Levine's work had a mixture of problem solving and systems (logistic) thinking.

Many theories reveal parallel processes between patient and nurse: conservation and adaptation (Levine, 1967); mirroring and mastering (Hall, 1966); and action and reaction (King, 1981). Orem (1985), in contrast, has one activity (self-care) but ownership of it shifts back and forth from patient to nurse.

It is interesting to note that Levine addressed two different contexts in her theory. In her earlier work, the explanation of structural and energy conservation was built on a context of disease, that is, the patient's condition is the basis. In contrast, her explanation of personal and social integrity was built on the context of the hospital (the negative aspects of being in an institutional setting). This reflects the tension many nurse theorists develop in trying to deal with normative physiologic data and unique, personal, humanistic information in the same theory.

SUMMARY

A complete theory includes not only clear definitions or descriptions of context, content, and process, but also provides the reader with an understanding of how these components interrelate. Context, content, and process provide a matrix, an organizing framework through which a theory can be understood or compared with other theories.

Table 2–1. *Comparison of Theories.*

Theorist	Content	Process	Context
Roy	Physiologic needs, self-concept needs, role function, interdependence	Nurse manipulates stimuli; patient responds to stimuli	Stimulus–response theory of human adjustment
King	Personal systems, interpersonal relationships, social systems	Patient and nurse: perception, judgment, action, reaction, transaction	Interpersonal systems
Orem	Self-care universals or health deviation self-care needs	Self-care by nurse, then by patient	Deficit in ability to do required self-care
Levine (early)	Structural integrity, energy, personal integrity, social integrity	Conservation by nurse; adaptation by patient	Problem solving
Johnson	Behavior systems (e.g., eliminative behavior or aggressive behavior)	Nurse manipulates behavioral responses, intervening through goals, drives, needs	World of human behavior
Rogers	Human field, environmental field, energy field, pattern, multidimensionality	Resonancy, helicy, integrality	World of continuously evolving man

A fourth element, goals, was not included in this discussion. Goals are the intentions that set direction and drive the entire theory.

Characterizing theories based on content, process, and context allows one to make simple comparisons among theories. Table 2-1 compares some of the major theorists in this manner. The reader will realize that some degree of accuracy and complexity has been sacrificed to achieve the comparisons.

REFERENCES

Brodt, D. E. (1980). A re-examination of the synergistic theory of nursing. Nursing Forum, 1, 85–93.

Chopoorian, T. J. (1986). Reconceptualizing the environment. In P. Moccia (Ed.), New approaches to theory development (pp. 39–54). New York: National League for Nursing.

Donovan, H. M. (1970). Toward a definition of nursing. Supervisor Nurse, 5, 12–15.

Finer, H. (1952). Administration and the nursing services. New York: Macmillan.

Hall, L. E. (1966). Another view of nursing care and quality. In K. M. Straub & K. S. Parker (Eds.), Continuity of patient care: The role of nursing (pp. 47–60). Washington, DC: Catholic University Press of America.

Johnson, D. E. (1980). The behavioral system model for nursing. In J. P. Riehl & C. Roy (Eds.), Conceptual models for nursing practice (2nd ed., pp. 207–216). New York: Appleton-Century-Crofts.

King, I. M. (1981). A theory for nursing: Systems, concepts, process. New York: Wiley.

Leininger, M. M. (1991). The theory of culture care diversity and universality. In M. M. Leininger (Ed.), Culture care diversity & universality: A theory of nursing (pp. 5–68). New York: National League for Nursing.

Levine, M. E. (1967). The four conservation principles of nursing. Nursing Forum, 1, 45–59.

Levine, M. E. (1971). Holistic nursing. Nursing Clinics of North America, 2, 253–264.

Levine, M. E. (1973). Introduction to clinical nursing (2nd ed.). Philadelphia: F.A. Davis.

Neuman, B. (1980). The Betty Neuman health-care systems model: A total person approach to patient problems. In J. P. Riehl & C. Roy (Eds.), Conceptual models for nursing practice (2nd ed., pp. 119–134). New York: Appleton-Century-Crofts.

Newman, M. A. (1979). Theory development in nursing. Philadelphia: F.A. Davis.

North American Nursing Diagnosis Association. (1989). Taxonomy I revised—1989: With official diagnostic categories. St. Louis, MO: Author.

Orem, D. E. (1985). Nursing: Concepts of practice (3rd ed.). New York: McGraw-Hill.

Peplau, H. E. (1989). Theory: The professional dimension. In A. W. O'Toole

& S. R. Welt (Eds.), *Interpersonal theory in nursing practice: Selected works of Hildegard E. Peplau* (pp. 21–41). New York: Springer.

Rogers, M. E. (1970). *An introduction to the theoretical basis of nursing.* Philadelphia: F.A. Davis.

Roy, C. (1980). The Roy adaptation model. In J. P. Riehl & C. Roy (Eds.), *Conceptual models for nursing practice* (2nd ed., pp. 183–187). New York: Appleton-Century-Crofts.

Rubin, R. (1968). A theory of clinical nursing. *Nursing Research, 3,* 210–212.

Strauss, A., Fagerhaugh, S. Y., & Glaser, B. (1974). Pain: An organizational–work–interactional perspective. *Nursing Outlook, 9,* 560–566.

Watson, J. (1988). *Nursing: Human science and human care: A theory of nursing.* New York: National League for Nursing.

Ziman, J. (1968). *Public knowledge: The social dimension of science.* London: Cambridge University Press.

3 The Normative Theory of Nursing

Before nursing leaders were cognizant of nursing theory as a domain for scholarly work, nurses and nurse educators still managed to work and teach effectively. Indeed, generations of nurses educated without reference to nursing theory perceived no shortcomings in their preparation. Despite the absence of a nursing theory, there was general consensus on what should be included in nursing education and what a nurse should and should not do in practice.

This chapter explores these shared expectations from the perspective of theory development. What is the unexplicated but shared theory of nursing that governs general practice? What are the generally accepted tenets around which nursing education and practice are structured?

It may be of value for the reader to brainstorm (as an individual or in a group) on these questions before reading further. Any nurse can easily come up with a list of precepts and rules that apply in nursing practice. The reader may be interested to see if she comes up with a list similar to that given in this chapter (derived from numerous classes of graduate students doing this exercise).

The objective of this exercise is to make the reader cognizant of the unstated expectations that influence the way in which a nurse goes about her work. These are the expectations that, if unmet, make a peer group question a nurse's performance. We will call these expectations *premises* of nursing practice. Because they underlie the way nurses practice, they constitute an operative theory of nursing, albeit uncodified.

The following values, beliefs, and operating rules are usually identified when a group of nurses examines the assumed bases of

Barbara J. Stevens Barnum: NURSING THEORY:
ANALYSIS, APPLICATION, EVALUATION, FOURTH EDITION.
© 1994, 1990, 1984, 1979 J.B. Lippincott.

nursing action. The first set concerns the nurse's beliefs about the patient:

> Pain is bad (except when needed for diagnosis); relief is to be desired.
> Anxiety is bad; a relaxed state of mind is to be preferred.
> Knowledge of one's condition and its management is to be preferred over ignorance.
> In most cases, knowledge of one's prognosis is to be preferred over ignorance or deception.
> Independence is to be preferred over dependence.

These patient-based premises underlie the actions and approaches taken by most nurses. They could be restated as nursing principles for action; for example, the nurse should relieve anxiety, the nurse should alleviate pain.

The next group of factors relates more specifically to how the nurse presents herself or how she acts. In these premises, the nurse

> never reveals repugnance for sights or smells associated with a patient, but masks any revulsion caused by putrefaction, vomitus, body excreta, or human disfigurement
> never displays unwillingness to serve the patient, but presents herself as pleased to render any legitimate service of whatever nature
> never reveals her own anxieties and fears, but presents a facade of professional control in all situations
> relieves the patient's embarrassment by dealing matter-of-factly with levels of intimacy that are unusual in other settings; for example, she assures the patient that his exposed body is routine for her and that he should not be embarrassed during her intimate care procedures
> provides reassurance as a basic mode of interacting with the patient
> always supports the patient's confidence in his physician, even when she has little personal faith in the particular practitioner
> always presents a positive outlook to the patient concerning his condition and its likely outcome, or toward his ability to cope with the resultant state
> establishes good rapport and positive interpersonal relationships with all patients
> encourages the patient to express his feelings
> treats the patient as a whole person instead of as just so many body parts, systems, or diseases
> tells the patient what she will do before she does it

works within the constraints of asepsis, accurate patient
identification, and coverage by physician orders where
required

bases her actions on her knowledge of pathology and of the
human body and its responses to illness and therapy

carefully monitors the patient's condition, reporting critical
changes to the physician as well as using them in nursing
decisions

provides body hygiene and implements therapies dictated by the
physician or by her knowledge of the patient's condition

preserves the functional capacities of the patient's body

works toward the patient's return to health with optimal retention
of his capacities or toward his peaceful and dignified death

The next set of premises has to do with the nurse's beliefs, values,
and expectations. The nurse

feels empathy, not sympathy, for the patient

expects the patient to acquiesce to her care

believes that cleanliness is a major virtue

suspends judgment of the patient, whatever his life-style and
background, and supports his inherent dignity

believes that illness and accidents, with the exception of some
life-style–related occurrences, happen to people
serendipitously and are not their fault

takes ultimate responsibility for her own actions, even for acts
done under physician's orders

believes that nursing is an art and a science

believes that nursing is a separate independent profession

believes the nurse has a moral obligation to her patient above all
others

This is not to say that the nurse always acts on these premises.
But when she breaks one, she is conscious that she is doing something
irregular. In so doing, she probably pauses to reflect and justify the
deviance to herself, if not to others.

ANALYZING THE INHERENT THEORY

If one assumes that these premises represent a theory of nursing,
how might one analyze them as a coherent framework? Obviously
they represent a helter-skelter set of values, rules for action, and
expectations—an ad hoc collection (descriptive theory) at best.

One way to analyze a theory is to explore the separate theory
parts. We will start in this fashion. One of the most arresting things
about these premises is the mixed values concerning honesty—au-

thenticity, if one prefers the existential term. There are pleas for honesty (the patient should be told his condition and prognosis, allowed to vent his feelings) along with masking of the nurse's own feelings (denial of the nurse's repulsion for certain sights, smells, tasks; denial of embarrassment on the part of the nurse; inculcation of empathy instead of sympathy). There may be outright dishonesty on the nurse's part in supporting the patient's faith in his physician, pretending confidence whether or not she feels it.

It is inconsistent for a theory to support values of honesty and dishonesty simultaneously. Often the honesty is required from the patient, the dishonesty from the nurse. The bifurcation of values—the discrimination between patient and nurse behaviors—is not unusual in theories, although many find it intellectually irresponsible when values and goals held for half the population (patients) are different from those for the other half (nurses).

Every theory of nursing must deal with two sorts of people: patients and nurses. The nature of this bifurcation is important in analyzing any theory of nursing. Indeed, some theories are contrived as if the patient and the nurse were creatures from different planets. Take, for example, a theory that explains man (the patient) on a biologic stimulus–response basis, yet describes the nurse as acting out of a psychological free-will orientation. Such a theory has an unjustified schism. After all, nurses and patients do come from the same root race. If the theory purports that patients operate on the basis of stimulus–response, there is no reason to assume that nurses function on a different principle.

The shift in the nature of man between patient and nurse often is more subtle than this illustration. Some theories see the patient in one context (for example, a biologic one) whereas the nurse is seen in another, the psychological perhaps. Another theory might describe the patient as a person involved in making health care decisions but simultaneously treat the nurse as the sole decision maker. The reader should always ask, Are the nurse and patient members of the same species? Do they function in same world?

Our normative theory of nursing, incidentally, is not irrevocably open to the criticism that a schism exists between patient and nurse. It *is* possible to envision a single race of people in which half are honest and half selectively dishonest. Nonetheless, it is a peculiar state of affairs.

Perhaps the most gracious thing that can be said about the deceptions advocated on the nurse's part is that they are aimed at making a difficult experience easier for the patient. An existentialist, of course, might find such deception difficult to justify.

Some theories of nursing claim to be based on existential principles advocating authenticity and honesty on the part of the nurse as well as the patient. Sometimes existential theories are advocated without consideration of how they conflict with present nursing practices. Consider the two conversations below, the first from the normative theory of nursing, the second from an existential perspective.

Normative Example

PATIENT: I'm sorry you have to do that, nurse. Irrigating a colostomy is revolting.

NURSE: It doesn't bother me at all, Mr. Smith. It's part of my job. I do this every day. You'll get used to it soon, and it won't seem so bad.

Existential Example

PATIENT: I'm sorry you have to do that, nurse. Irrigating a colostomy is revolting.

NURSE: It's distasteful, but it has to be done. Once you're used to it, it won't be quite as unpleasant.

In most cases, the second example would be more honest, but even the nurse who claims to want authentic existential relationships with patients may—because of her indoctrination in the norms of nursing—have difficulty in being true to her principles. Yet a consistent existential perspective does not call for authentic behavior only when convenient.

The dictate that approves of empathy but not sympathy is a related aspect of the normative theory. The advice may be symptomatic of other distancing tactics recommended to the nurse (e.g., masking disgust or embarrassment). Even the nurse's uniform and professional status may be seen as distancing strategies. Here, we find a tension between creating distance from the patient versus establishing rapport (another dictate of the normative theory). It is unlikely that both can be achieved simultaneously. Which is best? Which is healthy? For whom—the patient or the nurse? But in demanding both distance and closeness simultaneously, the normative theory can be accused of holding incompatible elements.

Another tension in the normative theory of nursing is that created by the difference between parts and wholes. Much of the education on which the nurse bases her actions (physiology, pathology, pharmaceutics) is founded on disciplines that compartmentalize man into parts. Yet she is expected to act toward man in a holistic fashion above and beyond a consideration of parts. Can one learn in one manner, yet act in another?

In the normative theory, there is a clear theme that positive emotions are supportive of health and recuperation (e.g., anxiety and pain are bad for the patient; the nurse maintains a positive outlook and offers reassurance, supports the patient's faith in his physician, and suspends judgment of the patient). This endorsement of positive emotions may remind the reader of Norman Cousins's (1979) advocacy of laughter as a cure for disease. To what degree does this aspect of the theory (positive emotions as curative) conflict with the simultaneous reliance on sciences such as pathology and physiology?

It is peculiar to note that when emotions are examined in nursing curricula (rather than inferred in normative rules), they are seldom explored as healing tools. Emotions are studied as feelings a patient has, not as tools the nurse uses. There is a disjunction between what the nurse is instructed to *do* concerning the patient's emotions and what she is taught *about* emotions.

In the normative theory, certain values are accepted with little examination. For example, independence on the part of the patient is always seen as a condition to be promoted. But what research has been done to test for therapeutic effects from periods of dependency?

The previously discussed aspects of normative theory are illustrative, not comprehensive. Notice, however, that we have approached the task by looking at one part at a time, or at a few parts as they interrelate. That is only the beginning of an analysis. Next we look at the theory as a whole.

THE THEORY AS A WHOLE

In analyzing any theory, one must view it as a conjoined set of elements to be considered in terms of balance and representativeness. One looks for what is missing as well as for what is present. From this perspective, the dictates of the normative theory focus heavily on values and emotive aspects of care.

In contrast, there is little attention given to methods. True, one finds obeisance to asepsis and cleanliness, but there is not much that could be termed methodology. For a profession in which much of the practitioner's time is spent in overt physical action, this is peculiar. The technology of bodily care (or principles directing it) is curiously absent from the list.

Even though most of the values and goals of the theory are emotive, there is little indicating what methods the nurse should use in achieving them. How does one care for a patient *as a whole*? How does one effectively *reassure* a patient? How does one *reduce anxiety*?

Sometimes use of the reflective question (a possible method for achieving affect-related goals) is included in the premises for the normative theory. In practice, the reflective question often turns out to be a device behind which the nurse hides to avoid answering awkward questions. The lack of premises concerning methods may not be as surprising as it first appears; indeed, it is reflected in the nursing literature. Consider, for example, the literature related to the nursing process. Great effort has been given to creating taxonomies of nursing diagnoses (intellectual labeling), whereas much less is written concerning methods of nursing intervention (practical hands-on care). Work on interventions currently is being addressed at the University of Iowa; that work is discussed later in this book.

Of similar interest is the focus on the nurse as monitor. Observing appears to be an important function in the normative theory. But monitoring, like diagnosing, is an intellectual act rather than something *done* to or for the patient. Only one premise in our theory deals with what use the nurse makes of the information gained in monitoring.

Another impression of the normative theory comes from the large number of prohibitions it contains. Many dictates concern what the nurse should *not* do rather than what she should. Is there a disempowering psychological effect from a focus on the negative? Indeed, numerous sociologists have commented on this negative aspect in nursing.

Other observations might be made concerning the normative theory of nursing, but we will not attempt to be comprehensive. Suffice it to say that,

- there is a general consensus concerning what should be done by nurses
- the premises can be examined together from a theoretical perspective
- they form an inconsistent pattern of ad hoc items, some of which are incompatible with each other

Furthermore, the list seems to be incomplete in terms of offering guidance regarding *methods* and *hands-on aspects* of nursing care.

In addition, the reader may wish to know that the premises selected for the so-called normative theory were the items most often volunteered by students in numerous graduate education classes addressing this topic. The same exercise with different groups of nurses might have produced different premises. The ones identified here, however, have been consistently identified by graduate nursing student groups.

NORMATIVE THEORY UPDATED?

The normative list offered in this chapter accumulated over a decade of asking students to reminisce on their education. But some elements may have fallen by the wayside in the hectic changes of the past few years. For example, I suspect cleanliness is no longer next to godliness. In fact, a patient is lucky to get a bath in many frenzied institutions. Another change I perceive involves blame. In many cases, the patient is made to feel responsible for his disease—more likely, ironically, if it is cancer than if it is alcoholism.

How has the normative theory of nursing changed over the past decade? The following section gives my personal impressions. I propose that nursing can be perceived as occurring through three different modalities of practice, each with its own approach. These modalities most closely relate to the settings in which the care is offered.

In hospitals, nursing has become care of the body. Indeed, we might think of acute care as the *body shop*. Here, homeokinesthesia is the game. The medical model reigns as nurses and physicians share patients, goals, and ideologies. Despite attempts to substitute nursing theories, I think that, on the whole, nurses in hospitals think in the medical model, using differential diagnosis or problematic thought, translating as needed to chart according to nursing models. See Chapter 4 for an illustration of this point.

Because patient acuity has intensified in the hospital, the body shop image has prevailed. Intensive monitoring of all body systems is possible and necessary given the heroic therapies used on people housed there. Ongoing adjustments in interactive body systems present a subtle dance of interventions, first with this system, then with that. It is these body systems associated with the medical model of man, not more esoteric nursing theories, that absorb the nurses' attention in the acute care setting.

For these acutely ill patients, nursing has become medicine, with monitoring/adjusting tasks in which the nurse either makes the adjustments or tells the physician exactly what is required. And the physician, if he is secure enough, providing the nurse was astute in her observations, will order what the nurse suggests. In essence, the medical model is alive and well.

With the radical human body insults, the intensive monitoring, and the invasive therapy required in this setting, I do not think it is a bad idea for nurses and physicians to be working with the same model. It certainly improves their ability to communicate.

The acute care setting is the one where it is most difficult to argue that medicine and nursing are separate and different professions. Nurse practitioner roles enhance this blurring across lines. Many nursing schools support the model of nurse as junior physician, whether they realize it or not. In these programs, course content is more and more practitioner oriented rather than focused on discrete clinical specialist knowledge.

The truth is that, in this highly technical practice, the caring interpersonal elements seldom come first in the nurse's mind. Indeed, the old activities associated with aspects of caring (such as bathing and feeding) are often done by bath aides, feeding specialists, and nurses' aides. In acute care today, the registered nurse primarily does advanced procedures, and I suspect that the theory most used is the medical model.

That is not the case in nursing homes, long-term care facilities, and home care. The interaction theories, the old public health models, and most extant theories of nursing can still be applied in these settings. Among others, Roy (1980), Orem (1985), problem-solving, man/environment models, and most constellations of the nursing process can be used in these settings and often are.

For one thing, the pace is slower—and by that, I do not mean that the caseload is lighter. But even when the nurse is swamped, she has time to mull over her care designs. Plus, she has fewer interactions with physicians and other health care workers and more control over her practice world. Indeed, it may be that this environment is more properly a nursing world.

As a matter of fact, the environment for home care and long-term care is similar to what existed in hospitals when most extant nursing theories were being formulated. The care given in homes and extended care today is what used to be offered in hospitals. In these settings, the nurse has the opportunity to think of the whole person; there is the luxury for a more comprehensive view of the patient beyond mere body work.

Where the body shop (acute care) was cell/organ/system oriented, the step-down level of care is more macroscopic: man in his environment. How does the patient with the recently fractured hip manage at home? Activities of daily living tend to be a major focus; family and community relationships get considered. Nurses in step-down environments often use a problem-oriented approach, whether they say so or not. A problematic approach works well in these environments and tends to be compatible with a holistic conceptualization of man. (Both holism and a problem-oriented approach are examined in detail later in this book.)

The step-down care environment is also the home of the middle-level nursing theory, partly because these patients tend to be sorted by kind. Geriatric care is a good example. Here, reinvolvement theories compete with disengagement theories, and bodily safety loses out to client peace of mind as quality-of-life issues modify care practices. The arena of step-down care is exciting, because its domains are of more interest to nurses than to physicians—arenas where it is more appropriate to consider the whole person.

The third nursing area deals with what I call mind–body work. Here, the nurse works with the well or vulnerable in the community, often in a private practice, in places of employment, or in community settings where groups come to seek enhancement of their health or quality of living.

The services offered in mind–body work range from exercise to smoking cessation to psychotherapy (often Jungian) to stress reduction. Psychosomatic is definitely not the descriptive word for these services because most of these mind–body ventures focus on wellness.

Nurses in these settings use the expansion, improvement, development theories, many laying claim to theories of Rogers (1970, 1990), Newman (1979, 1986), or Parse (1981). One hears of chakras, energy, therapeutic touch, spirituality, wellness, and life-style, and one hears of practices such as those of Krieger (1981) and Quinn (1984, 1989, 1992). And—yes—some of the caring theories, such as Watson's (1979, 1988) and Leininger's (1988, 1991), creep in.

In the mind–body work, the theory often is developmental, usually highly personal versus the public health/community orientation of step-down nursing. Psychotherapy, acupuncture, holistic healing, meditation, guided imagery—many newer techniques prevail in this arena. This is where many entrepreneurial nurses cluster, with both clinical nurse specialists and nurse practitioners often in private or collaborative practice.

RELATIONSHIP OF NORMATIVE THEORY TO NURSING THEORIES

One may speculate concerning how much the normative theory of nursing affects nurses ostensibly using other theories of nursing. We described earlier the difficulties that the normative theory presents for a nurse attempting to act from an existential base. The existential theory is not the only theory that might clash with the normative theory. Some holistic theories of nursing claim that the nurse need not know the patient's medical condition or disease state to do good nursing. This stance conflicts with the normative premise rooting nursing in knowledge of the biologic sciences.

The normative theory also conflicts with growing sentiment concerning personal responsibility for disease and illness. Some newer theories claim the individual, on some level, chooses his degree of illness or wellness.

It is surprising that nurses educated using various theories of nursing are still able to work together efficiently and effectively. They are able to evaluate each other's work and generally agree on whose practice is excellent and whose is poor. This speaks to some underlying agreement concerning what nursing is all about.

Let us look for a moment at the behavior of two nurses using different theories, those of Orem (1985) and Johnson (1980). Suppose that on sequential days these nurses are assigned to the care of the same patient: a young woman, in deep coma with extensive cranial trauma, on a Stryker frame because of additional spinal cord injuries.

The two nurses would do just about the same things for the patient, albeit with subtle differences. Even the differences, however, might be due to personal style as much as nursing theory. Surely neither would let the patient's eyes remain open without lubrication; neither would neglect skin care; neither would ignore fluid intake and output ratios; neither would allow dependent edema to accumulate in tissues if it could be prevented; and neither would neglect to test for changes in the woman's level of consciousness.

These nurse behaviors are easily explained by Orem's theory of self-care. The nurse using Orem's theory is simply substituting for the self-care the woman would provide for herself if she were able. It is more difficult to justify these actions on the basis of Johnson's theory—a theory in which the nurse intervenes in patient behavioral systems. Indeed, the woman's behavior, so far as we know, is highly limited. This is not to say that Johnson's theory could not be turned and twisted to fit the case; indeed, it could.

The issue is whether the theory is turned and twisted to fit what the nurse perceives needs to be done anyway, or whether the theory effectively dictates what she should do. Is the nurse's action dictated by some implicit normative theory? Is the purported theory (Johnson's) simply an overlay?

This is not a criticism of Johnson's theory; there are numerous cases in which Johnson's theory would be an effective basis of care. And there are numerous cases in which Orem's theory would have to be twisted and turned to fit the facts of the case. The issue is whether a normative theory of nursing underlies what all nurses actually do with patients. If there is such a normative theory, it is time that we define it more adequately. If we could capture the theory of extant practice, we would have an excellent basis for improving it. And it would be a challenging opportunity to work with an *is* theory as opposed to an *ought* one.

Another possibility is that, as nursing theories develop, they may become more discrete concerning what nursing acts their followers will perform. Then greater differences in practice may appear than is presently the case. Perhaps, eventually, a customer will select nurses holding to one theory over nurses using another, the same way he selects today among physician, osteopath, and homeopath.

SUMMARY

It is important to keep in mind that nursing theory should direct a practical set of activities directed toward specific goals. One way of keeping an eye on the essential linkage between theory and practice is to periodically examine how nurses practice, asking what tenets, values, and directives undergird what nurses actually do and think.

Are these values and dictates consistent with those expressed in our formulated nursing theories? If not, either the theories or the practices should be brought into consonance. Ultimately theory must be reality-based if it is to serve us. Looking at the notions that control the practice of any era is a first step in formulating or evaluating theories.

Looking at practice through theory-colored glasses also enables us to see changes from era to era, from one practice setting to another. Behind all examination of extant practice rides the teasing question: Is there an unstated but accepted theory of nursing that is prior to and basic for the theories that are advocated in the nursing literature? And, if so, how can we tease the theory out so that it may be clarified and examined?

PRACTICE EXERCISE

Just as one can derive a tentative nursing theory from familiarity with practice (as was done in this chapter), it is possible to infer a model of nursing from written works that address nursing practice. Select a nursing specialty journal. Choose three clinically based articles from the same or different issues. (Do not pick articles about nursing theory or sociologic factors of practice.)

Read the articles concerning clinical practice through "theory-colored glasses." Then see if you can describe how the practitioners of the specialty view nursing from a theoretical perspective. Make a brief list of premises that were stated or could be inferred from the articles.

A cautionary note: Usually journals choose similar pieces, but now and then you may find a journal that prints radically dissimilar articles. If this happens, compare and contrast the nursing worlds represented by the articles rather than try to conjoin them. If another nurse reads the same articles, you will benefit by comparing your reflections. Do not compare notes, however, until you both have analyzed the nursing works independently.

REFERENCES

Cousins, N. (1979). *Anatomy of an illness*. New York: W.W. Norton.

Johnson, D. E. (1980). Behavioral system model for nursing. In J. P. Riehl & C. Roy (Eds.), *Conceptual models for nursing practice* (2nd ed., pp. 207–216). New York: Appleton-Century-Crofts.

Krieger, D. (1981). *Foundations for holistic health nursing practices: The renaissance nurse*. Philadelphia: J.B. Lippincott.

Leininger, M. M. (Ed.). (1988). *Care: Discovery and uses in clinical and community nursing*. Detroit, MI: Wayne State University Press.

Leininger, M. M. (1991). The theory of culture care diversity and universality. In M. M. Leininger (Ed.), *Culture care diversity & universality: A theory of nursing* (pp. 5–68). New York: National League for Nursing.

Newman, M. A. (1979). *Theory development in nursing*. Philadelphia: F. A. Davis.

Newman, M. A. (1986). *Health as expanding consciousness*. St. Louis, MO: C.V. Mosby.

Orem, D. E. (1985). *Nursing: Concepts of practice* (3rd ed.). New York: McGraw-Hill.

Parse, R. R. (1981). *Man–living–health: A theory of nursing*. New York: Wiley.

Quinn, J. F. (1984). Therapeutic touch as energy exchange: Testing the theory. *Advances in Nursing, 6*, 42–49.

Quinn, J. F. (1989). On healing, wholeness, and the Haelan Effect. *Nursing & Health Care, 10*, 552–556.

Quinn, J. F. (1992). Holding sacred space: The nurse as healing environment. *Holistic Nursing Practice, 4*, 26–36.

Rogers, M. E. (1970). *An introduction to the theoretical basis of nursing*. Philadelphia: F.A. Davis.

Rogers, M. E. (1990). Nursing: Science of unitary, irreducible, human beings: Update 1990. In E.A.M. Barrett (Ed.), *Visions of Rogers' science-based nursing* (pp. 5–11). New York: National League for Nursing.

Roy, C. (1980). The Roy Adaptation Model. In J. P. Riehl & C. Roy (Eds.), *Conceptual Models for Nursing Practice* (2nd ed., pp. 179–188). New York: Appleton-Century-Crofts.

Watson, J. (1979). *Nursing: The philosophy and science of caring: A theory of nursing*. Boston: Little, Brown.

Watson, J. (1988). *Nursing: Human science and human care: A theory of nursing*. New York: National League for Nursing.

4 Basic Assumptions Underlying Current Nursing Practice*

IMPLIED THEORY

In Chapter 3, we looked at some of the general normative elements of nursing theory. Here, we will put this sort of reflection to work in an actual nursing practice situation. In Chapter 1, I discussed the fact that much nursing theory is based on what ought to be rather than what is. This chapter tries to remedy that.

Extant nursing practice is an interesting place to start if we are to shape theory effectively, because clinical practice is where nursing knowledge is grounded and extended. Nursing knowledge should shape our theories, and then, reciprocally, theories should direct our practice. If a nursing theory is to be any good, it must be practical. If we cannot evolve theories that truly direct practice, then we are wasting a lot of time with theoretical issues.

Even today, not all nurses view nursing theory as a vital component of practice. Perhaps this is because of deficits in our present theories, or it may be an inability on our part to convey the utility of the theories we have formulated.

True, knowledge should arise from practice; it should fold into theory, and theory, in turn, should inform practice. Theory, knowledge, and practice should fit naturally together; in most disciplines they do.

---

*Much of the material in this chapter was first presented at the Conference on Knowledge Development in Nursing, College of Nursing, Rhode Island University, Kingston, RI, September 26, 1991.

Barbara J. Stevens Barnum: NURSING THEORY:
ANALYSIS, APPLICATION, EVALUATION, FOURTH EDITION.
© 1994, 1990, 1984, 1979 J.B. Lippincott.

In disciplines that do not admit to having a theory—such as medicine—it is interesting to see what occurs when new ideas conflict with the *implied* theory. American medicine's early resistance to acupuncture is a case in point. Acupuncture meridians ignored known nerve paths, contradicting the cellular, organ, system theory that forms the basis of the medical model. No doubt this theoretical incompatibility slowed acceptance of acupuncture despite careful records of its effectiveness.

How does nursing theory relate to the actual work that nurses or nursing students do? Although Chapter 3 looks at this question from the armchair perspective, the cases illustrated in this chapter are a result of my own observations and those of my graduate students.

The reasons I look at extant practice are twofold. First, you have to know what is happening today—*right now*—before you can say it needs change. Then, if you do not like what you see, it is easier to change something you *know* than to work in a vacuum.

As is mentioned in Chapter 3, no matter what theory a nurse claims to follow, she is likely to do approximately the same things as other nurses when placed in the same work situation. When you think about it, that is truly remarkable.

Is it possible that so many different nursing theories lead to identical actions? If we were to look at another field—say psychiatry—it does not work that way. A Freudian psychiatrist, a Jungian, and a Skinnerian behaviorist would do very different things with the same client. Their approaches would be unique, their goals distinct.

Yet in nursing there is much uniformity in the actions of nurses espousing different theories. Do all roads really lead to Rome? Do all the different theories and rationales truly result in the very same actions? Or with greater development will the various nursing theories prescribe more variation in practice than is the case today?

Are our theories rationalizations designed to work backward to a set of acts intuited on a more basic level? Are the nursing theories we have devised actually in service to some overarching but still unrecognized theory of nursing practice?

The descriptive approach—looking at what nurses actually do—has never been popular with nurse theorists. All of our general theories, from Roy (1980) to Orem (1985) to Paterson and Zderad (1988), tell what the good nurse *ought to do*. If it isn't somebody's notion of *good* nursing, well, it isn't nursing.

Despite this strong bias, as a teacher, I assign doctoral students to observe hands-on nursing in various settings—a loose, grounded theory approach. The objective is to have them look at what actually happens and see if, from observing extant nursing acts, they can infer a theory of nursing underlying the practice. It is hoped that they can do this without imposing a ready-made value system on the observations, without being blind to the things one might not *want* to see.

It is true that not every observer approves of what the nurses do, but at least the method offers hope of developing a baseline on nursing practices. And, in most cases, analysis proves that the nurses were actually working to some end, in some sensible fashion.

STUDENT FINDINGS

I learned a lot about nursing attitudes in my early work with such observations. I remember, for example, when a class of six doctoral students—each observing independently in diverse settings such as intensive care, nursing clinics, nursing homes, coronary care—all came back with similar findings.

From those observations, five of the students wrote a scholarly paper entitled "Avoidance and Distancing: A Descriptive View of Nursing" (Flaskerud, Halloran, Janken, Lund, & Zetterlund, 1979). What had impressed this particular group of students was that all the nurses observed used strategies to build space between themselves and their patients.

The approach the students took to analyze this behavior was the one we had used in class; we asked, If the nurses create space between themselves and their patients, what function does this behavior serve?

I look back on the resultant paper with particular interest in the present era, when notions of caring and authentic relationships undergird so many nursing theories. So much is written about the necessity for a close nurse–patient relationship, so little about the function that distancing serves.

The most interesting lesson of this particular student endeavor was that most of the major nursing journals rejected the article, usually with rejoinders that nurses "shouldn't" be distancing themselves from patients. It was a strong message about nursing theory: Do not tell us *what is* unless it matches our ideal expectations. *Nursing Forum* finally published the article—the only journal that would take a chance.

Over my years of teaching, I have continued with observation groups and focus groups, giving nurses the opportunity to explore the commandments that operate in their minds when they give care. Because my classes were made up of graduate students, I had groups of bright contemporary practitioners.

The nurses who were observed never had trouble identifying the dictates of their nursing practice. Ask the right question at the right time and any nurse can explain why she did X instead of Y or Z. Often these operating dictates had little to do with espoused nursing theory.

PERSONAL OBSERVATIONS

The rest of this chapter describes the last time I personally followed a student nurse at practice. I have no reason to think this day was atypical. My account gives an overview of the relationship of theory and nursing practice as it occurred that day.

The senior student nurse I observed was assigned to a medical unit of a typical acute care hospital. She came on duty at 7:30 A.M., got report from the head nurse, and was assigned to two patients. The first, Mrs. Jones, was a 68-year-old woman who had suffered a myocardial infarction 5 days earlier. She had been released from the coronary care unit only a day ago and was still on cardiac monitoring. In this particular hospital, the monitor could be read from the patient's room or the nurses' station.

The second patient, Willie, had cirrhosis of the liver and had gone into renal failure. He had been on the unit about 1 week, was on intravenous (IV) fluids with more or less normal output, but was still receiving peritoneal dialysis every 6 hours.

The problem with Willie, so the head nurse said, was that the doctors wanted to get him off vasopressors, but every time they tried, his blood pressure dropped. At present, they were trying again to maintain his blood pressure by an IV drip of normal saline, no vasopressors.

I found it interesting that the head nurse called one patient Mrs. Jones and the other, Willie; the student nurse adopted those labels, so I will use them here to retain the flavor of the day. Although I had no doubt that the name differences reflected an unrecognized social bias, Willie got the lion's share of the nurse's attention. Both Mrs. Jones and Willie received various medications, by mouth for Mrs. Jones, IV for Willie, except for a vitamin by mouth.

The student checked on Willie first. He seemed to be sleeping but when she talked to him, he opened his eyes and answered coherently. When she quit asking questions, he drifted back into a mild stupor. She took his blood pressure: it was in the low nineties. She immediately went to the head nurse to report it. The head nurse said, yes, it was low, but they were trying to wean him from vasopressors—just watch it and try to stabilize the pressure by regulating the IV fluids.

The student went back to the room, speeded up Willie's IV drip, then looked at his output bag. Obviously, it had occurred to her that if she ran the fluid too fast, Willie would diurese, defeating the purpose of building up blood volume to increase blood pressure.

She drew a halt to her zeal, slowed the drip a little, making it slightly faster than it had been when she first entered the room but slower than her first instinct. Although we did not discuss her action, I am certain that her knowledge of the interplay of fluids with the body systems was the source of this correction. This was the start of the balancing game of the day—to keep Willie from going into shock because of low blood pressure, to keep him from diuresing, yet avoid administering the vasopressors that would lend artificial support to the blood pressure.

The student watched Willie like a hawk—his vital signs, his level of consciousness, his blood gases and oxygenation. It was a fine act in achieving equilibrium, and she adjusted the IV flow time after time. Several times, she notified the head nurse because the pressure slowly but surely fell. Each time, the head nurse said simply to keep watching it.

The student's attention to Mrs. Jones involved giving her pills. (Both patients had been bathed by a night bath team.) The student asked Mrs. Jones if she had any pain, and Mrs. Jones said, "Yes, the small of my back is killing me."

The nurse nodded and said, "Let's change the angle of the bed and see if that helps." She cranked the bed up a notch or two. I think it is safe to say this was a token effort more than an expectation that it would bring relief. If the patient had complained of heart pain, I am certain the student's efforts at pain relief would have been more substantial.

The student did not ask Mrs. Jones any other questions once she knew the patient had no heart-related pain. She reassured Mrs. Jones that she would be available, "if you need anything."

She then checked to make certain the cardiac monitor was attached and working, being sure it would bleep in case of a problem. In essence, the machine monitored Mrs. Jones while the nurse monitored Willie.

The student nurse made no attempt to increase her involvement with Mrs. Jones, but then her mind was on the balancing act with Willie. I am certain that situation would have been different if Mrs. Jones had any symptoms of heart failure, but she did not.

The student was particularly worried about Willie's status when she let the peritoneal dialysate run into the abdomen. While the fluid was indwelling, she checked his blood pressure every few minutes, and again when the fluid was released.

Ironically, the only time all day that the nurse relaxed was when the physician finally ordered vasopressors. This did not occur until Willie's blood pressure drifted into the low eighties. Once medication was given, Willie's blood pressure immediately went up to 110, and the nurse breathed a sigh of relief.

It might seem strange that the only time the student was at ease all day was when the physician admitted failure and resorted to drugs, but that is the way it was. This may serve as a humbling reminder that what is best for the patient is not always best for the nurse.

Then what? At the end of the shift, the student—who had been recording medications, treatments, and vital signs all day—went to a well-worn photocopy of nursing diagnoses hanging on a chain in the nursing station. She leafed down until she found a couple of diagnoses that would allow her to say the things she wanted to write. She put the diagnoses into the nurses' notes, followed by her comments. She did not go through the rest of the list to see if there were any other diagnoses she should have addressed; she also had not consulted the list in planning or executing her day's work.

In charting on Mrs. Jones, she did not mention the back pain Mrs. Jones had complained about three times during the day. The last two times the nurse had said, "That happens when you're in bed this many days." The nurse then went off shift to a clinical conference with her instructor. At this conference they discussed the student's patients based on Watson's (1988) carative theory of nursing, the model used by that particular school.

THEORETICAL CONCLUSIONS

So what is the point? This student ran into two theoretical structures for nursing that day. Let us look at the school's theory of caring. Had the student acted out of that model? Well, she gave care in two senses. First, she was *careful* in monitoring both bodies. True, she relied on the cardiac monitor for Mrs. Jones, but that left her free for the more complex monitoring required by Willie. Yes, she was careful in the sense of cautious or guarding—but that is not exactly what Watson's notion of caring is all about.

The nurse also expressed care in the sense of *taking care of*, in that she followed medical orders, gave pills, ran dialysate, recorded vital signs. Yet this is not the primary sense of caring in Watson's theory either.

One might debate whether she *cared* about either patient in the aspect of care called concern, emotive affect—the notion closest to Watson's theory. It was clear that the student turned Mrs. Jones aside with platitudes rather than expressed any sense of caring concern. Yet what would the student have done if Mrs. Jones sensed a willing ear and unloaded her anxiety? The student really was not free to be with Mrs. Jones in that caring sense. (I realize this is casting the student's performance in the best light possible, and she could be faulted for ignoring the patient's back discomfort, let alone discouraging the unasked questions that might have surfaced with the slightest probing.)

But the student's mind was constantly with Willie. It might have been worse if she had offered tidbits of false interest to Mrs. Jones when she was not prepared to follow up on them.

Did she express caring concern for Willie? When she was about to do anything, she always told him clearly, and he looked up from his mild stupor and said, "Okay." Beyond this, the student showed no overt signs of emotional attachment—no pat on the arm, no squeeze of the hand. Should she have worked harder at expressing her concern—assuming she had it? What would it have gained?

I think the clearest concern shown by the student was her fear that Willie's low blood pressure would bring on a major crisis and endanger his life. Yet I have little doubt, from her many pleadings to the head nurse, that she was far more interested in removing the possibility of this threatening scenario than she was in weaning Willie from reliance on vasopressors.

I was tempted to go to that clinical conference. If the student did not *care*, affectively, for Willie all day long—I am not saying she did not; I just could not see it—I suspect that she expressed plenty of concern when she gave her report to the instructor. It also seemed to me that a caring attitude might have evoked more concern for Mrs. Jones's backache. I cannot help but think that the caring theory had almost nothing to do with her actions in the clinical arena.

The second, and one might think more pertinent, brush with nursing theory occurred when the student had to base her charting notes on the hospital's system of nursing diagnosis. The charting format allowed the nurse to chart only after listing a diagnosis to which her comments related. In this particular use of nursing diagnosis, there was a lengthy battered list from which she might choose. (It was clear that other nurses thumbed the list daily.)

Now one might say these nursing diagnoses were important to the student's activities except that she never consulted the list until the end of the day. It was a retroactive effort in which the student hunted until she found a diagnosis that would allow her to say what she wanted to say anyway. The diagnosis was in no way directive of her practice; it was a structure into which she crammed her thoughts after the fact.

This nursing theory element had an impact on practice, if not the expected one. It became one more obstacle impeding nursing practice—the student could not talk about Willie until she put her thoughts into one of the dictated categories.

Now this does not mean that I am against the use of nursing

diagnoses, but I think a *good* theory should have helped the student during the work of the day—not later when she had to chart. A good theory should be practical; it should direct practice.

Did our student practice all day without any theory? I do not think so. I think she had a theory in mind, and I think it was the medical model of cellular, organ, and system function. And I do not think it was a bad model, given the two patients in her care.

The whole problem with Willie was to maintain a delicate balance among failing systems. The patient had deficits in at least three critical systems—renal, liver, and circulatory—not to mention the resultant deficits in his levels of consciousness and cognition. Frankly, if Willie were part of my family, I would prefer that she worry about his systems rather than focus on affective involvement—if she had to choose.

What about the second patient? It may well be that Mrs. Jones was ready—even ripe—for a caring relationship. But it was also clear that this student was not prepared to offer it because of the time and attention demands created by Willie.

No doubt the care given to Mrs. Jones was minimal, deficient from any notion of comprehensive care. But at least the student made sure the cardiac monitor was attached and working. Are there theories that would have allowed the same focus on vulnerable body systems while adding a more sensitive expression of concern? Why did she seem so little affected by the model promulgated in her school?

We may decry the medical model, but I think it was alive and well in this particular student's practice that day. It was the only theory I know that could account for all the student's activities that day.

Let us look for a moment at the nursing process, with its conjoined list of diagnoses. Supposedly, this construct directed practice on the unit. The question is whether it was truly directive or whether the nurses worked backward from a medical model orientation to this construct. If nursing process is applied retroactively instead of guiding practice, it is ineffective.

If an imposed model is not followed, that is not always bad. Nurses are not stupid; given a chance they will seek a directive structure that works most efficiently. If I did not have faith in their intelligence, I would not be interested in inferring theory from observed practice.

One may argue that the student ignored the unit's theory of practice because it conflicted with her school's carative model. It is true that students often find themselves in this double bind. In the case of this student, that argument would have been more compelling if she had used the carative model—but she did not.

From my observations, I think it is safe to say that students are wonderfully creative in subverting all curricular and practice-setting impediments that get in the way of their learning. The question becomes, What do nurses really learn about giving care, and where and how do they learn it? And, to what degree—if any—are the theories they learn directing or even modifying that care?

Are the caring theories too global? Do they fail to give the nurse a basis for her actions? Does the nursing process/diagnosis formulation suffer from the opposite fault—presenting an overwhelming number of pieces (process steps and diagnoses)? Can the nurse really consider all the available diagnoses (i.e., respond to each one that possibly fits a patient)?

The nursing student I observed did not use either of these theoretical models. Instead, she worked on a system of differential diagnosis applied to a cellular, organ, system notion of man—in other words, the medical model.

Some might protest that the nursing process is the same as the medical model, but that is not true. In most systems using nursing process and nursing diagnosis, when a nurse assesses her patient, she is supposed to identify all the applicable nursing diagnoses.

In contrast, when a physician assesses a patient, he does not run through the latest classification of accepted medical diagnoses. He does not work his way down the alphabet of diseases, written or mental. "No, the patient doesn't have Addison's disease; no, he doesn't have a brain tumor, or Cushing's disease, or dyspepsia either."

The physician does not consider all the possibilities; instead, he works by the method of differential diagnosis—branching logic instead of checking out a whole world of possibilities. Starting with whatever he recognizes as aberrant, the physician uses a thought pattern something like this: If it's a tumor, is it cancerous or benign? If cancerous, is it operable or inoperable? If inoperable, is it amenable to therapy *A* or therapy *B*? Instead of tracing out all possible diagnoses, he follows a trail of decision making through a process (called operational thought) that makes either/or choices at each step, ignoring and dropping other aspects of the model.

In the nursing process model, this is usually not the suggested format. Most who use the process recommend that a nurse start with *all* the applicable diagnoses, implying that the nurse should consider the whole model at one time. In this application, nursing is giving support to a system of great complexity. To return to the case of our student, did we foster nursing theories that were interesting but simply did not work? Was the fault in the systems? In the student? In the conflict between models to which she was exposed?

Nurses fall back on systems that work when it comes to actual patient care. This student nurse, if my perceptions were accurate, used a medical model. And I would have difficulty asserting that she was wrong, given her assignment.

In all our nursing theories, we have eschewed use of the medical model. The reason is self-evident: nursing is trying to prove its independence from medicine. Should we take a fresh look at the medical model? Is it the best choice in certain situations, with certain patients? Can it be modified or adapted to meet nursing requirements?

More important, is the medical model the hidden model underneath all our rhetoric? The student I observed had learned it somewhere. I am not advocating that nursing return to a medical model; I am simply saying that—like any other proposition—it should be analyzed for its fit and effectiveness in practice. Any theory, including the medical model, should be treated with similar dispassion.

Notice that this student's behavior (failing to use models she *ought* to use) was not unlike the situation in which my other students identified the principles of distancing and avoiding. In both cases, unpopular notions reared their heads in actual practice.

As long as we let an ingrained value system keep us from examining unpopular notions—such as avoidance, distancing, and the medical model—we have not gained the psychic distance necessary for dispassionate evaluation. Something is lacking in our intellectual honesty when the behaviors demonstrated by nurses at work are judged and found wanting before being given due consideration.

Finally, the reader is advised to peruse the work of Benner (1984), who did a masterful job of looking at nurses in practice in relation to how they think on the job. In her work, she examined thought processes as they related to experience and found that nurses' ways of thinking change over time. For example, the thought processes behind the nursing process may apply better on lower levels of expertise than on higher ones.

Should practice become the basis for all theory generation? Not necessarily. But it should not be overlooked as a testing ground for our notions of theory. Some of our best theorists are those who approach their own practice with a questioning manner and an open eye.

SUMMARY

This chapter has carried forth on the notion expressed in Chapter 3, namely, that practice and theory should inform each other, that theory should be practical and directive of actual practice. Notice that in a brief day's observation I saw instances of conflict between practice and theory as well as instances where the nurse probably wasn't aware of the theoretical basis for many of her actions.

While it is easier to see inconsistencies as a "removed" observer, there is no reason why a practicing nurse cannot learn to think about such issues during her own practice.

Notice that one of the obstacles to a nurse's thinking about what she is doing and why is the set of dictates she brings to her work, the set of values popular at any historical moment. In this particular case, the notions that a medical model and avoidance behaviors are "bad" may have been responsible for creating blinders.

Additionally, differences between the philosophies of a school and a practice arena may have placed a special burden on the nursing student in my observation. This problem deserves serious attention by faculty and practicing nurses in clinical settings where students are expected to perform.

REFERENCES

Benner, P. (1984). *From novice to expert: Excellence and power in clinical nursing practice*. Menlo Park, CA: Addison-Wesley.

Flaskerud, J. H., Halloran, E. J., Janken, J., Lund, M., & Zetterlund, J. (1979). Avoidance and distancing: A descriptive view of nursing. *Nursing Forum, 2*, 158–174.

Orem, D. E. (1985). *Nursing: Concepts of practice* (3rd ed.). New York: McGraw-Hill.

Paterson, J. G., & Zderad, L. T. (1988). *Humanistic nursing*. New York: National League for Nursing.

Roy, C. (1980). The Roy adaptation model. In J. P Riehl & C. Roy (Eds.), *Conceptual models for nursing practice* (2nd ed., pp. 179–188). New York: Appleton-Century-Crofts.

Watson, J. (1988). *Nursing: Human science and human care: A theory of nursing*. New York: National League for Nursing.

5 Touch or Technology: The Tension in Today's Nursing Theory

DICHOTOMIES IN NURSING

Each era brings a different tension to the subject of nursing theory. At one stage, the argument—with strong proponents on each side—was whether or not nursing should have a theory. That argument settled, nurses in schools and practice arenas contended with their peers in selecting the best theories for their practices. Next came the great press for universal agreement on a highly favored theory, namely that of the nursing process. Advocates and opponents of this method brought nursing theory to a new phase of political intrigue.

At present, the tension is a standoff between two highly disparate philosophies (and their related theories). The two camps can be captured in short by Naisbitt's (1982) coining of the opposing ideologies of *high touch* and *high tech*. Let us look at how these contrasting philosophies have affected health care and nursing in particular. Later, we will examine the specific theories that have attached to each position.

In the practice environment, be it hospital, home care, or long-term care facility, growth is toward increasingly high-technology practice. In contrast, many educational programs are dominated by high touch, often with curricula centered around one or another theory of caring. In part, the choices reflect the differences in environments. In the complex, highly demanding service setting, there are times when practicing nurses feel too busy, too pressured, to tend to the patients' needs for human concern (high touch in Naisbitt's

Barbara J. Stevens Barnum: NURSING THEORY:
ANALYSIS, APPLICATION, EVALUATION, FOURTH EDITION.
© 1994, 1990, 1984, 1979 J.B. Lippincott.

terms). In today's health care environment, some nurses cope by tending the machines rather than the patients.

Given the complexity and high demands of the intricate life-preserving/monitoring machinery, it is easy to understand this failing. Coping by distancing, we would say, if a patient did it. At its worst then, high tech may be a flight from the emotive demands of an environment in which patients are sicker and sicker, technology ever increasing, at the same time that nursing resources are stretched thinner and thinner.

In contrast, many educators have taken the opposite flight from complexity. Overwhelmed by the machines, by the rapid turnover of procedures and equipment, uncertain of how such complex and changing practices can ever be taught, some faculties have selected theories located in nursing's soft underbelly. These educators stress emotive principles, often located in nursing's caring theories.

This is not to call either caring theories or technical advancement wrong. They become wrong only when they are advanced *against*, and to the exclusion of, the opposite dimension. Where this occurs, the pattern represents flight from difficult realities. The truth is that the needs for high technology and high touch are both present in all caregiving environments. The philosophic problem is that these two notions seldom rest comfortably within the same theory.

In light of the passage of time, it is interesting to go back to the origin of high tech/high touch as coined by Naisbitt (1982) in *Megatrends*. By now, most people have adopted his terms but have forgotten what he said about them. Naisbitt forecast the dichotomy but saw the technology as inevitable, unstoppable. High touch, he said, would develop as a rebellion to it:

> A very poignant example of what I mean by high tech/high touch is the response to the introduction of high technology of life-sustaining equipment in hospitals. We couldn't handle the intrusion of this high technology into such a sensitive area of our lives without creating some human ballast. So we got very interested in the quality of death, which led to the hospice movement, now widespread in this country (Naisbitt, 1982, p. 42).

It is clear that nurses and other health care workers have created backlash movements as Naisbitt predicted. This does not mean that these movements lack inherent value. No one would deny the importance of the hospice movement, for example. But that does not lessen the accuracy of Naisbitt's prediction.

REACHING EQUILIBRIUM

What was Naisbitt's solution to the dichotomy between high touch and high tech? He called for a balance, a notion that needs careful consideration. How does one balance high tech/high touch in the modern health care facility? One does not do it by ignoring the machines and teaching only an affective attitude of caring nor by performing high-tech skills but ignoring human needs.

Naisbitt's solution was *balance*, not an either/or choice. But what sort of balance is required? Obviously, the higher the technology, the greater the need for the compensating high touch. This is the problem not yet solved by extant nursing theories. The higher the technology, the greater the need for the compensating high touch.

A patient wired to three beeping machines in an intensive care unit is more in need of high touch than is the patient receiving less technologically imposing care. Striking the right proportion requires excellence in both domains simultaneously. The caretaker must have the technologic skills *and* the human element of caring. Neither alone is adequate. The truth is that increased technology has not only made the techniques of nursing practice more complex, but it has also made the need for high touch more intensive.

IDEOLOGIES ASSOCIATED WITH HIGH TOUCH, HIGH TECH

In theoretical terms, a problem arises when trying to serve goals of high touch and high tech simultaneously. The problem is that these two notions arise in competing ideologies about the world and the patient.

In theoretical terms, we call this *context*. You may remember that in Chapter 1 we identified context as different from content, process, or goals of a theory; it forms the background on which a theory plays out. Let us look at the patient to highlight the difference between high tech and high touch.

The patient to whom high tech is applied is primarily a physical body, expected to react like most other physical bodies. The neurologic, chemical, and physical aspect of body are the targets of the high-tech strategies. The therapeutic interventions are designed to bring these elements of being into conformity with desired norms.

In contrast, the patient to whom high touch is applied is the individual in his personhood, the human separate from all other persons. High touch concerns the person as he expresses his unique needs, desires, will, and emotions. These aspects of personhood clearly affect health but cannot be programmed; they are not amenable to high-technology intervention.

Biofeedback might be considered a technique that, to some degree, bridges from person to body, from high touch to high tech. Similarly, some uses of imagery may cross the line. Take the case in which a patient with cancer is told to imagine his healthy cells destroying the aberrant ones. On the whole, the interface between person and body is a new area of exploration, despite older wisdom concerning psychosomatic disease. Even the term *psychosomatic* brings to mind a state in which the psyche works negatively, incurring a disease condition. In psychosomatic medicine, one attempts to change the behavior and patterns of affect as part of the cure. For example, one tries to induce a Type A personality to adopt a more relaxed attitude toward life postmyocardial infarction, or one attempts to get a patient with ulcers to decrease his exposure to stress. But more radical therapies that bridge the psyche–body gap are just coming onto the scene.

NURSING THEORIES: BLENDING HIGH TOUCH, HIGH TECH?

In nursing, some theories address both person and body, touch and technology. The issue is whether they do it effectively or whether they address two contexts instead of one. Consider Levine's (1971) theory as presented in Chapter 2. Conservation of energy and structural integrity deal with man as biology, whereas conservation of personal and social integrity deals with man as a person. Some would argue that her later work (Levine, 1973) bridged this contextual difference by applying homeokinesis to both aspects of man.

The popular nursing process, and its related taxonomy of nursing diagnoses, favors the high-technology side of the equation. Even though some of the diagnoses might be psychological, the inference is that the process is so scientific that it is "removed" from the personhood of the nurse. Supposedly, any group of intelligent nurses studying the same patient would come up with the same diagnoses. The system calls for application to all patients of routinized assessment tools (the patient's history, physical examination) to reveal self-evident conditions. The assumption is that the diagnoses are logical conclusions, external to the nurse, conclusions that are *in fact* evident in the patient.

This removed, technical theory contrasts with notions of nursing arising from the caring models. In these models, the personhoods of both nurse and patient are involved, making human interactions unique, not replicable. In most of these theories, caring is an emotion the nurse brings to the situation by virtue of how she feels, not a tool she carries with her like scissors.

In essence, nursing's move toward theories of caring may be seen as a reactive stroke to the high tech of our provider environments—just as Naisbitt predicted. But we must go the next step and realize that the backlash alone is not a solution. Successful nursing depends on blending and balancing high touch and high tech in equal measure, and we must find a way to bridge these opposites in our nursing theories.

It is not surprising that some schools and practices have opted for either/or positions, because the task of teaching and performing both aspects may seem overwhelming. These are the horns of today's theory dilemma. It is interesting that, in the past, the contrast of these two elements led to a notion of technical versus professional nursing, in which *professional* came to mean does not know the technology but is an expert in nurse–patient interpersonal relationships. In this constellation, the baccalaureate-prepared nurse recognized the patient as a person and responded to his human needs, whereas the associate degree or diploma nurse provided the techniques of care.

Making high tech/high touch the dividing line between levels of nurses was not a tactic that ever worked effectively. Vice-presidents of nursing practice complained vociferously that baccalaureate graduates could not function in the care environment. Furthermore, as the technology grew, right or wrong, status tended to accrue to the technologically skilled—not a situation designed to be compatible with the nursing image. More recently, differences among professional and lower-level nurses have been located in the levels of decision making rather than in a high touch/high tech separation.

There is, of course, a natural order in the education of students. Only when the technology is second nature will the nurse be secure enough to focus on high-touch aspects. Until her hands know what they are doing, she probably cannot attend to the patient's human need for caring.

Is there a nursing theory that gives equal time to these two principles? Probably not. As indicated in Chapter 4, the medical model certainly is compatible with a high-technology environment. And, as claimed earlier in this chapter, the nursing process with concurrent taxonomies of diagnoses and (just coming on the scene) taxonomies of nursing interventions is also compatible with a high-technology ideology. This is so because the patient is seen as a case that is "out there," apart from the nurse who inspects and treats him. The attempt is to create a level of scientific certainty concerning the patient, his deficiencies and their treatments. The theories supporting a high-tech ideology are those that come down heavy on the science side of nursing.

In contrast, the theories that support a high-touch orientation either favor the view of nursing as an art or attempt to explain science in radically new ways. Most theorists label these as *caring* theories.

Thus, high tech is captured in theories that devise a "one system fits all" process focusing on the science of nursing. In contrast, high-touch theories focus on interpersonal subjectivity between nurse and patient.

Although there are no theories that purport to hold high tech in itself as their base, there are middle-level theories based on notions of touch. Ironically, even among theories of touch, there are some that exemplify the science or technology side, others that fall on the high-touch side. Let us examine both kinds.

THEORIES OF TOUCH

At first glance, the term *touch* would appear to be the same as Naisbitt's high touch, but the situation is not that simple. Naisbitt's concept of high touch concerns caring more than physical contact, and some theories of touch go the opposite direction.

Touch: even this finite form of caring is not simple. As Weber (1990) has said, there are several unique notions of touch: to be in contact with, to communicate, and to lay hands on.

The first meaning (contact) might best represent a physical–sensory model, typical of an Anglo-American philosophy, according to Weber. The second (to communicate) is associated with European existential and phenomenologic models, whereas the third (laying on hands) comes closer to a field model and possibly an Eastern philosophy.

Nursing has done research on touch in all three paradigms. Consider the work of Diamond (1990). She explored the thesis that tactile stimulation improves central nervous system function (p. 73). This work, discussing mammalian forebrain responses to varied environmental conditions of touch, documents chemical and structural modifications in nerve cells.

Diamond's work illustrates Weber's first sort of touch: a physical–sensory model. In essence, this meaning of touch crosses the line into the high-tech ideology. Notice that Diamond talked about nerve cells, not persons; stimuli and responses, not human values or perceptions. Weiss's (1992) work also focused on the physical–sensory model (with some crossover to other ideologies), evolving a model interrelating qualitative and quantitative dimensions of touch, including location of touch, divided into 19 body areas; actions, divided into 28 gestures; duration, measured in seconds; intensity, measured in four levels; and frequency of contact, within specified time frames (p. 34).

Much of the work on touch in nursing resides in Weber's second ideology, a phenomenologic meaning, in which touch is seen as human communication. Take Fanslow's (1990) discussion of the elderly:

The human need for touch on all these levels does not lessen as we grow, develop, and age. Rather, the need for touch on all levels increases with age and wisdom. Physical, psychological, and emotional touches are all essential for the proper establishment of internal sources of security, self-image, trust, and interdependence (pp. 542–543).

In this view, touch is both bodily and mental. Sympathetic communication and meaning pervade the notion.

Therapeutic touch is the best example of Weber's final category. Krieger (1981) is the first name among nurses in this particular ideology. Krieger viewed therapeutic touch as having a direct effect on the human field, providing a manipulation of human energy fields. Krieger also saw therapeutic touch as having the potential for cure as well as for care (pp. 146–147).

To make the domain of touch even more complicated than the three senses defined by Weber (all of which have been incorporated into nursing), Leininger (1988) made us aware that touch also has a social meaning—one that may vary from culture to culture (p.18).

As a theoretical construct, touch has been adapted to both high-tech and high-touch philosophies. It may be that work such as Diamond's serves as a bridge between those two worlds. One can touch emotionally as well as physically in our common language. Diamond's work has purported a scientific physiologic need for touch, a need shared by all people alike. Leininger represents the opposite pole, showing how touch means different things in different cultures. Like Naisbitt's theory, the ultimate solution will not be either/or but both.

LOOKING AHEAD

Although touch is a narrower concept than caring, we can anticipate that the larger concept will have diverse meanings, too. We noted that the need for caring increases as technology expands. From a theoretical perspective, few if any of our nursing theories handle the two elements of high touch and high tech with equal competency. Achieving high tech and high touch is a major challenge for our era; the answer will require looking at our educational and service practices anew. It will involve questioning and revising old patterns, letting go of some cherished beliefs and strategies.

What can we do to bring high tech/high touch into proper balance in our professional practice? The goal is a worthy one and achievable. One approach views high touch as contextual, as a caring concern, an attitude of human warmth and sympathy. And attitudes are caught, not taught. If faculty and nursing managers show caring concern in everything they do, the attitude will be assumed and copied by students and staff. In this pattern—high touch as context—it becomes something to be demonstrated in performance, not subject matter for a lecture.

In this tactic, high touch is an essential part of the background in which care occurs. There is no need to increase course content hours or work hours. Instead, the context is manipulated, the image of how one behaves is conveyed by teachers and leaders as they go about the other aspects of nursing.

High touch does not always require the nurse to sit down at the patient's bedside and talk. Caring can be expressed—and felt—while her hands are busy with other things. There is no excuse for a nurse to say, "I was too busy to be caring." Caring should be evident in every aspect of her work—hands-on tasks included.

In this interpretation, staff learn that the attitude of caring is an expectation, not something the lack of which may be excused by a harried environment. It occurs simultaneously along with all task completion.

Because attitudes are caught, leaders must be careful not to damage the positive attitudes that students bring to the profession. Most students enter nursing to "do good" for people. But many soon learn that affect is less significant than scientific dispassion. Students are covertly discouraged from being warm caretakers when praised only for their scientific rigor—for their success in adopting a scientific, removed, disinterested attitude. This is not to say that the science of our craft should be neglected, but the caring element cannot be discouraged either.

ANOTHER OPTION

If, on the other hand, the caring aspect develops its own "technology," it may be necessary to divide nursing into component specialties rather than preparing a person for all sorts of nursing practice in a single program. If techniques such as therapeutic touch require their own schooling, it may be that one profession cannot encompass all that is required. In Chapter 3, we looked at the differences in care ideologies between acute care, step-down care, and well care. It may be that different sorts of nursing will develop, each specializing in its own techniques.

Some aspects of caring technology are breaking off already in the formation of curricula for healers. Many of the students in these schools and classes are nurses, but this profession-in-its-infancy is not developing as a subcomponent of nursing.

The notion of care as a unique technology of its own—the high tech of high touch, if you will—is discussed in the next two chapters.

SUMMARY

High touch/high tech is one of the latest in a string of dichotomies that has marked the history of nursing. Other dichotomies have included science versus art, technical versus professional, care versus cure, clinical specialism versus nurse practitioner models. Several solutions have been offered to such dichotomies over the years.

Sometimes the profession tries to handle a dichotomy by picking one side over the other. The selling of care over cure is one such historical example. Such a solution is two-edged, setting a clear and precise boundary around the profession, but limiting its growth as well. In essence, the boundary may pinch later. See, for example, Chapter 19, in which some theorists try to advance clinical specialism by ruling out advanced nurse practice as misplaced medicine.

Sometimes the profession solves a dichotomy by trying to have it all. When theorists assert that nursing is a science and an art, we see this solution in effect. Unfortunately, this solution may become a slogan rather than a carefully determined strategy and rationale. Few nursing theories, for example, have explained just how this particular opposite pair (art and science) can be combined successfully.

In other cases, the solution is to subsume one end of the dichotomy under the other. In the next chapter we will look at theorists who handle the care–cure dichotomy this way, by subsuming cure under a larger, encompassing concept of care.

We have not always picked the best solution in handling our dichotomies. Sometimes the choice has been narrow or self-serving, but seldom should we throw out one element without careful consideration of the consequences. The high touch/high tech dichotomy demands a successful resolution. In this chapter, I have suggested that choice of one side to the exclusion of the other has potential negative consequences for the profession. That does not mean that a resolution encompassing both principles will be achieved easily.

REFERENCES

Diamond, M. C. (1990). Evidence for tactile stimulation improving CNS function. In K. E. Barnard & T. B. Brazelton (Eds.), *Touch: The foundation of experience* (pp. 73–96). Madison, CT: International Universities Press.

Fanslow, C. A. (1990). Touch and the elderly. In K. E. Barnard & T. B. Brazelton (Eds.), *Touch: The foundation of experience* (pp. 541–557). Madison, CT: International Universities Press.

Krieger, D. (1981). *Foundations for holistic health nursing practices: The renaissance nurse.* Philadelphia: J.B. Lippincott.

Leininger, M. M. (Ed.). (1988). *Care: Discovery and uses in clinical and community nursing.* Detroit, MI: Wayne State University Press.

Levine, M. E. (1971). Holistic nursing. *Nursing clinics of North America, 2,* 253–264.

Levine, M. E. (1973). *Introduction to clinical nursing* (2nd ed.). Philadelphia: F.A. Davis.

Naisbitt, J. (1982). *Megatrends: Ten new directions transforming our lives.* New York: Warner Books.

Weber, R. (1990). A philosophical perspective on touch. In K. E. Barnard & T. B. Brazelton (Eds.), *Touch: The foundation of experience* (pp. 11–43). Madison, CT: International Universities Press.

Weiss, S. (1992, Spring). The tactile environment of caregiving. *Science of Caring, 2,* 32–40. (Available from School of Nursing, University of California, San Francisco, CA 94143.)

6 Nursing: The Care Ideologies

TRADITIONS OF CARING: ONE OF MANY PROPOSED BASES FOR NURSING

Many nurse theorists say that caring is at the heart of the profession. This chapter looks at that long tradition. What do our theorists mean by caring when it is used as a hallmark for nursing? How does that stance differ from other theories of nursing? More important, how do theories of caring differ from each other?

There is general agreement that nurses are caring people; most are drawn to the profession for that reason. That most act in a caring way is different from asserting that the *act of caring* is at the heart of professional nursing practice. In the past few chapters we looked at two models, the nursing process and the medical model, that would place the locus of nursing in a science of diagnosis based on examination and assessment of the patient.

We also referred to theories that find the nexus of nursing in other locations: Levine in conservation, King in transactional agreement on goals, Roy in manipulating stimuli toward desired responses, Johnson in the realm of behavior. All of these theorists would wish their nurses to be kind, but that is not the point. Caring happens in context; it is on the side—like french fries.

The theories we will look at next are different and growing in popularity—possibly as the backlash Naisbitt indicated. Many of the theorists holding caring theories are newer on the scene; their writings have been published more recently than the theories used so far as illustrations. And, some would say, their theories are more in keeping with the changing paradigm by which the world around us is understood—but more about that later.

Barbara J. Stevens Barnum: NURSING THEORY:
ANALYSIS, APPLICATION, EVALUATION, FOURTH EDITION.
© 1994, 1990, 1984, 1979 J.B. Lippincott.

DEFINITIONS OF CARING

Nurses are not in agreement concerning just what *caring* means. The ambiguous term *caring* (sometimes shortened to *care*) has at least three discrete meanings. The first has to do with taking care of in the sense of tending to another, doing for someone else. "Taking care of" tends to be expressed in physical acts meeting patient needs. The nurse takes care of the patient in tending to his bodily needs, just as the mother takes care of her infant. Care (or caring) in this sense of the word will be called *taking care of* in this chapter.

Orem's self-care has much of this sense to it. In this usage, care is a shorthand word for the doing of requisite tasks. We can label this sort of care as an *activity*. In the earlier discussion of high touch and high tech, the first requirement for a nurse was that she be at ease with the equipment and procedures. Taking care of, in this sense, may be closer to high tech than to high touch; at least it has to do with effectiveness in doing for another.

The second notion of caring has to do with a concomitant emotion or attitude that occurs in the nurse in relation to the patient. The nurse who cares is one who has an emotional investment in the patient's welfare; that is, she cares about him.

Caring, instead of *taking care of*, is used to indicate this meaning, namely, the case in which the nurse has a positive concerned feeling for the patient. We can label this definition of caring as *attitudinal* or *emotive* in contrast to the first meaning that we labeled as an *activity*.

Because it is possible for a nurse to take care of a patient with a caring attitude, the difference between these two meanings is sometimes lost. Yet the notions are separable intellectually and in practice: it is possible for a nurse to *care* but fail to *take care of*, as in the concerned nurse who sympathizes with an anxious patient yet fails to pick up the clues to his internal hemorrhage or fails to provide a needed, relaxing body massage. In the opposite case, it is possible for a nurse to *take care of* a patient's needs, using exacting nursing techniques, but still feel no real concern for him.

There is yet a third sense of care, that of *caution*, of being careful to do something correctly. Usually this sense carries a sense of guarding against injury or accident. Here, care has to do with caution or precision in one's acts. In this sense of care, the word *careful* seems most appropriate. Like the preceding notion of caring, this one is an attitude, but it is a *mind-set* rather than an emotion. Notice that all three senses of caring may occur simultaneously. A nurse may take care of a patient, with a caring attitude, and be careful to ensure that she does things in a safeguarding manner.

CONFUSING MEANINGS OF CARE

Confusion among the three meanings of caring is evident from early on in the nursing literature. In a classic theory piece, Kreuter (1957) begins with *caring*, but encompasses the notions of *taking care of* and *careful* as well:

> The word "care" has precise meaning. It belongs to the intellect and its root is in "sorrow." Care is not akin to cure. It is more related to "pathos" in that the feelings are touched. When one gives care, the feeling is experienced and responded to by extending oneself toward another. Care is expressed in tending to another, being with him, assisting or protecting him, giving heed to his responses, guarding him from danger that might befall him, providing for his needs and wants with compassion as opposed to sufferance or tolerance; with tenderness and consideration as opposed to a sense of duty; with respect and concern as opposed to indifference (p. 302).

Kreuter's slippage was an easy mistake; many others have made the same error. One reason is that all three principles of caring have importance in nursing; it is hoped that all three are evinced simultaneously in a nurse's practice.

In a modern discussion, Styles (1982) purposely combined two senses of caring:

> Despite our periodic raillery about the word "nursing" and the perceived stigma attached to this designation, our occupation is well named. Nursing is nurturing, nourishing, fostering, caring. Nursing is caring: both the attitude and the activity. Nursing is caring by promoting health and self-reliance for all. Nursing is caring for those who need to be nurtured in relation to their health status, whenever, as long, as frequently as they need it, until that need is removed or revised by recovery, independence, or death. This caring responds to needs ranging broadly between the extremes of information and incentive for maintaining wellness to emotional support and technical assistance for sustaining life and providing comfort. As nurses, our MOTIVATION is caring; our SERVICES are caring and managing; our fundamental TOOL is knowledge, both tacit and explicit; the PRODUCT of the services is health—its maintenance and restoration to the highest possible level of attainment—and physical and psychological comfort (p. 231).

Some modern theorists, concerned about cloudy meanings, have attempted to operationalize their definitions of caring. Gaut (1986) gave this definition:

> To state these requirements in another way, any action may be described as caring if, and only if, the carer (S) has identified a need for care and knows what to do for X (the one cared for); S chooses and implements

an action intended to serve as a means for positive change in X; and the welfare of X or what is generally considered as good for X is used to justify the choice and implementation of the activities identified as caring (p. 78).

Although Gaut's definition might still give us pause concerning the exact meaning of caring, her decision to relate caring to competency reveals that she is using the action-oriented taking-care-of form. Indeed, this form is easier to capture in an operations definition because it ends in an overt action.

The emotional, concerned meaning of care is harder to pin down. Authors seldom analyze the nurse's caring in this emotive form, nor do they usually interpret it as an act of will; instead, they see caring as a predisposition. Gaut, in contrast, called caring an intentional human enterprise—in other words, taking care of.

Usually one can rely on an author to mean care as *taking care of* when speaking about nursing behaviors; after all, this is action oriented. But even here we find an exception. Wolf (1986), like Gaut, talked about care as nurse behavior. When we look at the content of the behaviors, however, it is clear that she actually identified representative behaviors that give clues to caring (concern). Wolf called this form of caring "attachment":

When attachment behavior is aroused in stressful circumstances, the attachment figure, the caregiver, terminates the behavior by touching, clinging to, or reassuring the person experiencing the threat of loss (p. 85).

These are behaviors all right, but they are not behaviors in the usual *taking-care-of* sense, because they reveal the nurse's concern, her emotional involvement. Using this perspective, Wolf developed a Caring Behavior Inventory, arriving at a list of caring behaviors. The 10 highest ranked are given here:

1. listening attentively
2. comforting
3. being honest
4. having patience
5. being responsible
6. providing information so that the patient or client can make informed decisions
7. touching
8. showing sensitivity
9. showing respect
10. calling the patient or client by name (p. 91).

Like Gaut, Wolf attempted to operationalize a discrete meaning of caring, but her job was trickier because she was identifying observable phenomena that stand as evidence of an affective feeling.

EXTENDED MEANINGS FOR CARING

Not all theorists have limited the common meanings of caring to three. Morse, Bottorff, Neander, and Solberg (1991) identified five conceptualizations of caring as:

1. a human trait
2. a moral imperative
3. an affect
4. an interpersonal interaction
5. a therapeutic intervention.

In addition to carefully differentiating among these meanings, they also analyzed common care theories on these dimensions (pp. 120–121).

Swanson (1991), who worked on a middle range theory of caring, identified five caring concepts:

1. knowing—centering on the one cared for
2. being with—sharing feelings, not burdening
3. doing for—comforting, anticipating, performing competently
4. enabling—informing, generating alternatives
5. maintaining belief—believing in, offering realistic optimism (p. 163).

One of the challenges in defining care has been to capture the affective responses that accurately reflect caring. This is what both Swanson and Wolf tried to do. Another major bias in caring has always been the promulgation of empathy as opposed to sympathy as a desired nurse behavior. Of course, the meanings of these terms have been manipulated from author to author to enable each to take a preferred position without changing terms.

One interesting study by Boyd and Munhall (1989), involving the concepts of reassurance and sympathy, identified the following seven mechanisms of reassurance:

1. giving factual information
2. providing physical comfort such as holding one's hand, touching, covering with a blanket
3. giving theoretical information, for example, explaining what is "normal"

4. supporting the client's power
5. being present, staying and listening
6. projecting a confident, calm manner
7. crying with the client (p. 65).

This is an excellent beginning in theory building, that is, capturing a concept in factual behavior. It would be interesting to see how this variable of reassurance relates to the variable of affective caring. Also interesting is that Boyd and Munhall discovered nurses projecting their own feeling into clients erroneously (p. 64), for example, seeing the client as a victim of unfortunate circumstances when the client had a different perception entirely.

PERSONAL PERSPECTIVES

I would like briefly to reflect on caring as I have observed it in relation to the three basic meanings of the term defined in this chapter. And I would like to do this from my personal experiences as a patient and as a family member of a patient. Let me start with the experiences in which I was a family member. Three private duty nurses stand out in my mind, each coincidentally, exemplifying one aspect of caring.

Nurse A was the *careful* nurse. She did the "orders," no more, no less. She was *careful* not to put herself in legal jeopardy. Everything was done on time, using correct methods (technologically advanced care was required). She made no attempt, however, to relate to the conscious patient, although she did identify herself and say what she was about to do before doing it. She saw no patient problems; yet as a family member, I could identify many. She made no changes or adjustments in the care plan, established no rapport. In my intuitive judgment, I did not think that Nurse A was a good nurse. *Careful* alone simply was not satisfactory. We requested that she not come back.

Nurse B was the one oriented toward *taking care of*, yet her motivations seemed to be intellectual, not affective. She was fussy about the professional markers; she liked to be called "Miss B" and protested when the patient tried to use her first name (visible on her name tag). This nurse did everything that was ordered with great proficiency. In addition, she searched for and remedied patient problems, seeming to enjoy the problem-solving activity for its own sake. Her *taking care of* certainly included the aspect of being careful without focusing on it. She did all the right things.

She was particularly good at negotiating working arrangements with an obstreperous patient. In justice, I had to say that her professional judgments were the best of the group discussed here. What she lacked was any sense of caring. Somehow I sensed—and so did my sick relative—that her work, comprehensive as it was, stemmed from a sense of professional pride, not from a motive of caring for the patient. Somehow, she enraged my family member even more than had the indifferent nurse. And, though I could not help but judge her work to be good, to be honest, I did not want her back either.

Nurse C, in contrast to the others, focused on *caring* in the affective sense. She really cared about the patient. She was not nearly as professional as Nurse B. She used her first name, wore a red sweater and moccasins, and was overweight. When she was not busy, she read *Cosmopolitan* or *Redbook*. But she saw and solved many patient problems because she was sensitive to the patient's reactions.

Some might dispute her professional judgments. She let an exhausted patient sleep, putting off blood pressure checks despite known erratic fluctuations. If she had asked me, I would have made the same decision, and it would have been motivated by the same thing: an emotional response to the patient.

My conclusions about caring based on these observations were simple. The effectiveness of the nursing act was greatly enhanced when the nurse (Nurse C) really cared about the patient. From the patient and family perspective, it certainly mattered more than any other factor in the care.

My own experience as a patient was more complex. The nurse who was most supportive, most caring in getting me through a life-threatening episode—and I truly felt her support as invaluable—was also the nurse who made serious errors, considerably increasing the pain I would subsequently experience. The caring? It mattered a lot. The errors in therapeutics? That mattered a lot, too.

Can caring be the basis of care? In my own mind, I am thrown back to the dilemma faced in Chapter 5. Care or technology? Can one have dominance? Perhaps the question is which matters most if both are given in competent measure.

THEORISTS ON CARE

Wiedenbach (1970) was one of the early theorists to appreciate the place of caring in nursing. She believed that the intention of the nurse was an important part of her effectiveness, that the same act done with caring and without caring could have a different outcome:

> It is the nurse's way of giving a treatment, for example, that enables a patient to benefit from it, not just the fact that a treatment is given him; and it is her way of expressing her concern—not just the fact that she

is present or speaks—that enables him to reveal his fears. The nurse's way of using the means available to her to achieve the results she desires in her practice is an individual matter, determined to a large degree, by her central purpose in nursing and the prescription she regards as appropriate to its fulfillment (Wiedenbach, 1970, p. 1062).

Thoughts and feelings, including reactions, are integral parts not only of what we do or say but also of how we do it. . . . The thoughts and feelings that precede and accompany each act are the less apparent parts of nursing; yet, because they set direction for each act, they are the real determiners of the results the nurse achieves (Wiedenbach, 1963, p. 54).

Wiedenbach analyzed the "invisible" act of caring, and found that it was a tool that could be used to the nurse's advantage, ensuring her successful practice. This insight started a line of theory development that continues today.

The secret of the helping art of nursing lies in the importance the nurse attaches to her thoughts and feelings and the deliberate use she makes of them as she observes her patient, identifies his need for help, ministers to his need, and validates that the help she gave was helpful. If she recognizes her thoughts and feelings, respects their importance, and disciplines herself to harness them to her purpose and her philosophy, not only will she enrich her nursing practice, but she will in all probability experience enduring satisfaction from the helping service she has rendered (Wiedenbach, 1963, p. 57).

What Wiedenbach called concern is what we label caring. And although she explored these feelings methodically—scientifically, if you will—this is not the way we usually think about the caring part of nursing. Rawnsley (1980) made a more modern plea in terms not unlike those of Wiedenbach:

If the nurse is to focus on the person rather than the syndrome, however, she must develop a healthy symbiosis of the art and science of nursing within herself. This calls for her to integrate cognitive, psychomotor, and affective skills in such a way that each contributes to and acts in the service of the others, while maintaining its own distinct properties. Identifying, learning, and eventually synthesizing the continually expanding base of knowledge and skills specific to each dimension constitute the science of nursing. The art of nursing consists of successfully incorporating all three dimensions in practice, as demonstrated in helping behaviors on behalf of patients (p. 244).

Like Wiedenbach, Rawnsley used the term *concern* in discussing caring. And, for Rawnsley, this concern is nursing's primary business. Adopting Wiedenbach's notion that the affective component can become a tool, Rawnsley (1980) went further, asserting that there can be a science of affect. As she said, "Yet we must comprehend the affective dimension in order to use it deliberately." (p. 245) Although some might consider these affective aspects instinctive (and unlearn-able), Rawnsley envisioned their use in a disciplined fashion, that is, as the science of the art of nursing.

> To relate to the emotional life of others, one must grasp the variety, the mystery, and even the contradictions intrinsic to the human condition. Perhaps awareness of this complexity is intuitive; and perhaps apprecia-tion of it can be cultivated under certain prescribed learning conditions (p. 245).

In her attempt to make a science of the emotional side of nursing, Rawnsley identified two affective concepts: promotive tension arousal and empathy. The first is tension coordinated to another's goal attainment. Helping, according to Rawnsley, is a function of the level of discomfort or tension a potential helper experiences witnessing the plight of another. Empathy is a vicarious emotional response to the perceived emotional tone of another, a transient internalization of what it is like to be the other without being over-whelmed by the identification—*metafeeling* in her terminology (Rawnsley, 1980, p. 245).

Rawnsley's strategy, to some degree, was to intellectualize feel-ings—perhaps a tricky endeavor. Can the emotional response survive under the microscope? Although Rawnsley strived to make a science of the emotions, Ellis (1969) pointed out the dangers of losing it:

> There is some danger of neglecting, or even rejecting, some of the tradi-tional, familiar components in nursing as we grow in our emphasis on science and research. One such component might be what is termed TLC—"tender loving care." This something or this concept, which some-one (it would be fascinating to know who) has tried to capture by a phrase, is nonscientific. We are not likely to do research on it. We do not have tools to measure it. Yet many nurses, as well as nonnurses, recognize it as an essential component in nursing for many patients (p. 1438).

New Paradigms

Watson (1988) is one of the recent theorists closely associated with the notion of caring. She has maintained that "caring is the essence of nursing and the most central and unifying focus for nursing prac-tice." (p. 33) She also has said that "care and love are the most universal, the most tremendous, and the most mysterious of cosmic forces; they comprise the primal and universal psychic energy." (p. 32) Yet she has admitted that some persons are caring, others uncaring, defining an uncaring person as

> insensitive to another person as a unique individual, nonperceptive of
> the other's feelings and does not necessarily distinguish one person
> from another in any significant way (p. 34).

Stressing nursing's tradition of caring, Watson defined caring as
a transpersonal value. She gave us a sense of how it feels when caring
is present and a taste of its absence as well:

> It is not so much the what of the nursing acts, or even the caring
> transaction per se, it is the how (the relation between the what and the
> how), the transpersonal nature and presence of the union of two persons'
> soul(s), that allow for some unknowns to emerge from the caring itself
> (p. 71).
>   . . . the degree of transpersonal caring (in this sense of unity of
> feeling) is increased by the degree of genuineness and sincerity of the
> nurse. If the recipient feels that the nurse is contriving the feelings and
> is "going through the process," trying to act upon the other's feelings,
> and does not feel within his or her self what longs to be expressed,
> resistance immediately springs up (p. 69).

Watson seemed to assume the nurse (perhaps anyone drawn to
nursing) will be a caring person. Yet perhaps it is a matter of degree,
because in other parts of her books, she has stressed ways to teach
better caring through helping the nurse to develop as a person. A good
question for Watson would be whether applicants to her program are
assessed for caring potential before being admitted. One might think
this criterion more important than the grade point average, if her
theory is to be applied consistently.

With her commitment to caring, Watson (1979) called her 10
theory content/process items (nurse behaviors) carative factors:

1. formation of a humanistic–altruistic system of values
2. instillation of faith–hope
3. cultivation of sensitivity to one's self and to others
4. development of a helping–trusting relationship
5. promotion and acceptance of the expression of positive
   and negative feelings
6. systematic use of the scientific problem-solving method
   for decision making
7. promotion of interpersonal teaching–learning
8. provision for a supportive, protective, and corrective mental, physical, sociocultural, and spiritual environment
9. assistance with the gratification of human needs
10. allowance for existential–phenomenological forces (pp.
    9–10).

Watson's list of carative factors escapes the three senses of caring previously described in this chapter because it includes aspects that can best be considered as character forming for the nurse. Indeed, it would fit better into the categories of caring identified by Hutchinson and Bahr (1991) in relation to the elderly: protecting (safety and surveillance); supporting (facilitating coping and normality); confirming (recognizing personhood); and transcending (prayer and spiritual focus). It is interesting that Hutchinson and Bahr were describing caring behaviors of residents, not nurses, when they arrived at these categories.

Watson (1988) has focused heavily on the spiritual subjective aspects of both nurse and patient:

> In transpersonal human caring, the nurse can enter into the experience of another person, and another can enter into the nurse's experience. The ideal of transpersonal caring is an ideal of intersubjectivity in which both persons are involved. This means that the value and views of the nurse, though not decisive, are potentially as relevant as those of the patient. A refusal to allow the nurse's subjectivity to be engaged by a patient is, in effect, a refusal to recognize the validity of the patient's subjectivity. The alternative to caring as intersubjectivity is not simply the reduction of the patient to an object, but the reduction of the nurse to that level as well (p. 60).

Watson's theory of caring would be classified as interactional according to the schema offered in Chapter 1 for determining the locus of a theory (the nursing act, the patient, or the nurse–patient interaction). The reader will recall that an interaction theory focuses on the relationship between patient and nurse rather than on either party or their discrete activities/perceptions.

King (1981) was used earlier to illustrate an interactional theory. In her case, the nurse and patient act, react, interact, and finally transact, that is, agree on a goal or goals. Although Watson's theory is located in interaction also, the nature of the interaction is quite different from King's. Her intersubjectivity is transpersonal, occurring in a larger context, beyond both patient and nurse. In this sense, we are reminded again of the principle of synergy. The reader interested in a fuller understanding of transpersonal psychology may wish to read Wilber (1979, 1980).

Watson's (1988) focus on the nature of the nurse is intimately tied to her conceptualization of disease as disharmony:

> Where there is disharmony among the mind, body, and soul or between a person and the world, there is a disjunctive between the self as perceived and one's actual experience, and there is also a felt incongruence with the person, between the I and me and between the person and the

world. . . .This incongruence leads to threat, anxiety, inner turmoil, and can lead to a sense of existential despair, dread, and illness. If prolonged, it can contribute to disease (p. 56).

Obviously, in a theory such as this, treatment of illness takes on a metaphysical transpersonal character. Caring cannot arise except as an event between two people:

The context for viewing the person and the nurse in the theory of trans-personal caring is in the moment-to-moment human encounters between the two people. The coming together of the two—one the caregiver and the other the recipient—comprise [sic] an event. An event connotes an actual caring occasion in which intersubjective caring transactions occur (Watson, 1988, p. 71).

Watson is not the only theorist to have described nursing in a new paradigm that reinterprets man and his place in the universe. Newman (1986) even titled her book *Health as Expanding Consciousness.* This theory and others like it are discussed in Chapters 7 and 8. Suffice it to say that Watson is not alone in viewing nursing through a changing world view that radically alters the notion of nursing as well.

A Cultural Orientation

Leininger (1991), another major care theorist, may, at first glance, seem to have done the same thing as Watson, but that is not the case. It is true that she considers the patient's world, especially in the sense of the culture in which he resides. But, unlike Watson, her perception of culture is more traditional. Of course, Leininger would agree that the patient is affected by whatever world view is held in his society. If and when a new paradigm is established as mainstream thought, then she would take that into account.

For now, it serves to call her perspective anthropologic: it looks at the individual as he is influenced by his culture. Her main objective is to care for the patient, not to reinterpret his world or his meaning in it. Leininger takes the patient's world as a given and asks how his perception of it impacts on his health and how care should be offered in light of his perceptions.

What she shares with Watson is that she has fused caring with another element: in Watson's case, a new paradigm of man and his existence; in Leininger's case, the patient's culture. As Leininger (1991) has said, "All human cultures had some forms, patterns, expressions, and structures of care to know, explain, and predict well being, health, or illness status. I held the care was not an isolated activity. . .." (pp. 23–24) She further tightened this notion, making care and culture indivisible:

> *Culture and care were synthesized as a construct entity that are tightly embedded into each other in order to explain, interpret, and predict phenomena relevant to nursing. This culture care was conceptualized and transformed into a nursing perspective to develop a body of new or distinct knowledge in nursing (1991, p. 24).*

In her care perspective, Leininger differentiated folk care systems and professional health care systems, noting that the linking of these care systems must occur if culture conflicts, noncompliance behaviors, and cultural stresses are to be avoided (1991, p. 37). Nursing, she has said, must consider people's emic knowledge, that is, the meaning their experiences hold for them. Etic care imposition—based on the caregiver's constructed representation of the empirical world—simply is inadequate. In her model, Leininger (1991) identified three modes of culturally congruent care:

1. cultural care preservation or maintenance
2. cultural care accommodation or negotiation
3. cultural care repatterning or restructuring (pp. 41–43).

These modalities of nursing care are devised in relation to the patient's world view, including aspects such as technologic factors, religious and philosophical factors, kinship and social factors, cultural values and lifeways, political and legal factors, economic factors, and educational factors (Leininger, 1991, p. 43). Obviously, Leininger's model is a complex one, but she has done a good job of making us sensitive to aspects of parochialism that creep into our usual theory derivations.

> *All too often, some health practitioners do interfere with cultural lifeways and beliefs of culture by their so-called interventions and lack of culture knowledge. Hence, the caring nurse generally wants to work with and be congruent with the norms and values of the culture (Leininger, 1991, p. 55).*

The vulnerability of Leininger's model is that it requires extensive knowledge of a secondary discipline: anthropology. As Leininger (1991) has indicated, the utility of the model depends on the skill of the practitioner in applying it (p. 56). Of course, one can argue that merely developing sensitivity to cultural factors—even unknown cultural factors—is an important start.

In light of a transcultural perspective, Geissler (1991) took an interesting look at the nursing diagnosis work of the North American

Nursing Diagnosis Association. The reader will not be surprised that she found the diagnostic set culture bound.

ANALYSIS OF CARE THEORIES

In analyzing care theories, I find the chief issues—and the chief problems—arise when caring (affective) is shifted from context to content or process. In this fashion, caring becomes not the *attitude* with which the nurse gives her taking care of, but *the care* itself. In essence, the objective becomes to deliver an affective message of caring.

Is this an adequate basis on which to poise nursing? If it is, how do we justify the fact that nurses also need to learn other things—such as regulating body fluids, skin care, and, yes, highly technical procedures? When caring becomes the content or the process of a theory, it is difficult to justify the tasks commonly conceived as composing nursing.

Some theorists, such as Watson, did an excellent job of justifying caring as content or process, but it usually involved seeing the world and health in radically new ways. These may be interesting ways—they may even represent a changing world view. But at this stage, the new paradigm is still a deviation from the way the world is experienced by most of the society that constitutes our patient populations.

What is the solution when the nurse's world view and the patient's differ widely? Does one try to convert a patient to a new vision? Some theories would see ill health as an opportunity for just such a conversion. Indeed, some would see this as a path to health.

The shift of caring into content and process also brings with it another problem. When caring is seen as context, it can be role modeled, caught rather than taught. When it moves front and center, then it becomes a subject for study and analysis. This moves us into models where affect itself is presented as content to be learned. Will affective caring survive in the nurse's breast if it is held too long under the microscope? These problems are not meant to negate the interesting theories of caring, because it is clear that caring is an important concept in nursing.

It is also true that when caring is merely context, it is vulnerable. It may get lost from sight. Roberts (1990) examined caring in midwifery in an attempt to prove the profession has not been coopted by the medical model. She found caring characteristics, such as presencing, being with, and virtue, alive and well (p. 69). Such important characteristics, she claimed, are seldom recognized, rewarded, or taught. It would be difficult to say she is wrong. Clearly, part of the reason these elements get overlooked is that they are less visible as context. Yet many birthing women have shown themselves sensitive to context. Why else select midwives over obstetricians? Caring theories, because they cover such a wide gamut of beliefs and designs, will probably force the student to confront and evaluate her own image of the world. Perhaps that is their greatest value. Caring theories differ as to what is meant by caring and whether caring is pure affect or a learned tool; whether caring is an art, a science, or both; and whether caring is tightly bound to another concept (such as culture or a new world paradigm).

SUMMARY

Caring is a general term that means many things to many people. At the very least, caring may be seen as having three discrete meanings:

1. physical acts involved in taking care of
2. cautionary, protective nurse behaviors
3. affective, emotion-laden concern for the patient.

Often nurse theorists use the term *caring* without being precise as to which meaning is implied.

Whatever the sense of caring, it is important to know whether it is seen as the content of nursing, a context in which nursing acts are performed, or a process by which nursing is delivered. Even when it is seen "only" as context, caring may have a radical effect on the achievement of nursing goals, as illustrated by Wiedenbach's observations.

In addition to these differentiations, the notion of caring may undergo subtle changes in meaning based on the other concepts in a given nursing theory. For example, when care is linked to culture, the notion is different from when it is linked to a new paradigm view of the world. Because caring is a popular concept at present, that is value-laden, it is important to recognize when it represents a mere slogan superimposed on a theory that actually has a different base.

Whether the popularity of caring will last remains to be seen. Already some authors are recommending its replacement by one or more concepts embedded in the patient, not the nurse. Alternatives such as comfort, security, decreased anxiety, and hope have been suggested. These alternatives make us aware that caring is a nursing phenomenon, not patient-based. Others would note that it evokes a patient-based response not possible in its absence. How might that patient response be labeled? Should the chief values in a theory rest in the nurse or in the patient? The notion of caring brings us back full circle to the nurse–patient dichotomy expressed in earlier chapters.

REFERENCES

Boyd, C. O., & Munhall, P. (1989). A qualitative investigation of reassurance. *Holistic Nursing Practice, 1*, 61–69.

Ellis, R. (1969). The practitioner as theorist. *American Journal of Nursing, 7*, 1434–1438.

Gaut, D. A. (1986). Evaluating caring competencies in nursing practice. *Topics in Clinical Nursing, 2*, 77–83.

Geissler, E. M. (1991). Transcultural nursing and nursing diagnoses. *Nursing & Health Care, 4*, 190–192, 203.

Hutchinson, C. P., & Bahr, R. T. (1991). Types and meanings of caring behaviors among elderly nursing home residents. *Image, 2*, 85–88.

King, I. M. (1981). *A theory for nursing: Systems, concepts, process.* New York: Wiley.

Kreuter, F. R. (1957). What is good nursing care? *Nursing Outlook, 5*, 302–304.

Leininger, M. (1991). The theory of culture care diversity and universality. In M. Leininger, (Ed.), *Culture care diversity & universality: A theory of nursing* (pp. 5–68). New York: National League for Nursing.

Morse, J. M., Bottorff, J., Neander, W., & Solberg, S. (1991). Comparative analysis of conceptualizations and theories of caring. *Image, 2*, 119–126.

Newman, M. A. (1986). *Health as expanding consciousness.* St. Louis, MO: C. V. Mosby.

Rawnsley, M. M. (1980). Toward a conceptual base for affective nursing. *Nursing Outlook, 4*, 244–250.

Roberts, J. E. (1990). Uncovering hidden caring. *Nursing Outlook, 2*, 67–69.

Styles, M. M. (1982). *On nursing: Toward a new endowment.* St. Louis, MO: C. V. Mosby.

Swanson, K. M. (1991). Empirical development of a middle range theory of caring. *Nursing Research, 3*, 161–166.

Watson, J. (1979). *Nursing: The philosophy and science of caring.* Boston: Little, Brown.

Watson, J. (1988). *Nursing: Human science and human care: A theory of nursing.* New York: National League for Nursing.

Wiedenbach, E. (1963). The helping art of nursing. *American Journal of Nursing, 11*, 54–57.

Wiedenbach, E. (1970). Nurses' wisdom in nursing theory. *American Journal of Nursing, 5*, 1057–1062.

Wilber, K. (1979). *No boundary.* Los Angeles: Center Publications.

Wilber, K. (1980). *The Atman project: A transpersonal view of human development.* Wheaton, IL: Theosophical Publishing House.

Wolf, Z. R. (1986). The caring concept and nurse identified caring behaviors. *Topics in Clinical Nursing, 2*, 84–93.

BIBLIOGRAPHY

Alvino, D. (1986). A caring concept: Providing information to make decisions. *Topics in Clinical Nursing, 2,* 70–76.

Bottorff, J. L. (1991). Nursing: A practical science of caring. *Advances in Nursing Science, 1,* 26–39.

Drew, N. (1986). Exclusion and confirmation: A phenomenology of patients' experiences with caregivers. *Image, 2,* 39–43.

Engles, N. S. (1980). Confirmation and validation: The caring that is professional nursing. *Image, 3,* 53–56.

Gantz, S. B. (1990). Self care: Perspectives from six disciplines. *Holistic Nursing Practice, 2,* 1–2.

Holden, R. J. (1990). Empathy: The art of emotional knowing in holistic nursing care. *Holistic Nursing Practice, 1,* 70–79.

Krysl, M. (1988). Existential moments of caring: Facets of nursing and social support. *Advances in Nursing Science, 2,* 12–17.

Kurtz, R. J., & Wang, J. (1991). The caring ethic: More than kindness, the core of nursing. *Nursing Forum, 1,* 4–8.

Leininger, M. M. (Ed.). (1988). *Care: Discovery and uses in clinical and community nursing.* Detroit, MI: Wayne State University Press.

Leininger, M., & Watson, J. (Eds.). (1990). *The caring imperative in education.* New York: National League for Nursing.

Moccia, P. (Ed.). (1987). *Nursing theory: A circle of knowledge* (2-part video program). New York: National League for Nursing.

Morse, J. M., Solberg, S. M., Neander, W. L., Bottorff, J. L., & Johnson, J. L. (1990). Concepts of caring and caring as a concept. *Advances in Nursing Science, 1,* 1–14.

Paternoster, J. (1988). How patients know that nurses care about them. *Journal of the New York State Nurses Association, 4,* 17–21.

Rawnsley, M. (1990). Of human bonding: The context of nursing as caring. *Advances in Nursing Science, 1,* 41–48.

Shiber, S., & Larson, E. (1991). Evaluating the quality of caring: Structure, process, and outcome. *Holistic Nursing Practice, 3,* 57–66.

Tanner, C. A. (1990). Caring as a value in nursing education. *Nursing Outlook, 2,* 70–72.

Valentine, K. (1988). History, analysis, and application of the carative tradition in health and nursing. *Journal of the New York State Nurses Association, 4,* 4–9.

Warren, L. D. (1988). Review and synthesis of nine nursing studies on care and caring. *Journal of the New York State Nurses Association, 4,* 10–16.

Watson, J. (1987). Nursing on the caring edge: Metaphorical vignettes. *Advances in Nursing Science, 1,* 10–18.

7 Nursing: An Alternate Cure Ideology

For many theorists, care, as opposed to cure, has been the critical factor in differentiating nursing from the practice of medicine. But not all nurses agree that cure is the private territory of medicine. More and more, cure is claimed as legitimate turf for nursing activities. We will look at cure theories in nursing after first looking at one nurse who radically opposed cure as nursing.

CURE: NOT FOR NURSES, PLEASE

Until recently, most nursing education programs assumed care, as opposed to cure, to be the convenient boundary line between nursing and medicine. For at least one theorist, supporting this dividing line held great importance.

Appendix A encapsulates the early philosophy of Lydia Hall (1968), a nurse who was anxious to differentiate between nursing and medicine and was convinced that cure belonged to medicine, not nursing. She was equally convinced (in the 1960s) that cure was impossible in chronic care, which happened to be the specialty of her institution as well as an arena of care then assuming major importance.

By differentiating care and cure, she carved out a large territory for nursing—all of chronic care. She envisioned chronic care as a nursing domain, one in which nurses would make the decisions, hiring physicians as needed for episodic cure needs. More important, she was able to bring off this vision in her facility.

In her era, Hall used the care–cure dichotomy to carve out an independent domain of practice for nursing. It is ironic that in our

Barbara J. Stevens Barnum: NURSING THEORY:
ANALYSIS, APPLICATION, EVALUATION, FOURTH EDITION.
© 1994, 1990, 1984, 1979 J.B. Lippincott.

era, nurses are struggling to pull down that very wall for the same purpose: to increase nursing's scope of independent practice.

The arguments that Hall (1968) used to differentiate cure and care were interesting then and still are:

> Nurses and others who work there (in hospitals) have got caught up in the CURE activities which are emphasized to the neglect of CARE, the kind that is essential in helping the patient get to the CORE of his difficulties through learning (p. 2).
>
> When I ask physicians why they have not opened schools for practical doctors, as nurses faced with a shortage opened schools for practical nurses, I get an academic answer to an academic question. The truth is that physicians have not needed to open schools and will not, so long as they have "professional nurses" to whom they can delegate more and more medical tasks and activities. We have become "practical doctors" and so we say to the public by our behavior that we prefer being potential painers and practical doctors to being comforters and nurturers (p. 1).

Hall was one of the most vehement protestors against nursing's assuming cure-related activities. One supposes she might have seen some merit in the recently failed, physician-backed plan for registered care technicians—if the terminology were changed to registered cure technicians.

CURE: THE SUBSTITUTION THEORIES

Loomis and Wood (1983) also considered the nurse's role in chronic care. But the era had changed, the nurse's position had shifted on the spectrum of care versus cure. These authors took the position that the nurse, indeed, is engaged in curing activities in just the same way as is the physician. Successful management of a chronic health deviation, they said, is the equivalent of cure, and that is within the legitimate realm of nursing practice (p. 7).

Loomis and Wood agreed with Hall that chronic health care was the domain of nursing, yet they drew different conclusions about the nurse's role. Hall contended that the nurse must avoid cure activities; Loomis and Wood, that what the nurse is doing is cure.

Patient teaching can be viewed as cure in many circumstances. Teaching the diabetic to regulate his own metabolism, as Loomis and Wood would assert, cures him to the extent that a chronic disease is curable, that is, to the extent that the condition is amenable to ongoing regulation. It is difficult to maintain that teaching the regulation of insulin, diet, and exercise is primarily a function of caring (affective). Indeed, when one thinks of patient teaching in the context of curing, it becomes clear why some physicians still feel threatened by nurses assuming teaching tasks.

Recently, more nurses have come to question the fit of care and cure as the appropriate boundary between medicine and nursing. One reason is that nurses, in various ways, have crossed the line into more and more cure work. The primary nurse practitioner is a clear case in point. Primary care practitioners can now be found in almost every domain of practice, from the traditional midwives, to pediatric practitioners, to numerous newer practitioner roles in adult health.

Primary care has become a major arena of nursing practice, despite the early philosophical problems it gave some theorists and nurse leaders. The fear was that the nurse practitioners would identify with medicine, not nursing. And, indeed, there was some evidence that it happened then, and—to a small degree—still may happen today. But on the whole, most practitioners think of themselves as nurses in specialized practice, not as physician extenders.

Indeed, the present trend in nursing education is to combine clinical specialist and practitioner roles at the master's level. If the trend continues, it will be difficult to find a traditional clinical specialist program in a few years. The question of care versus cure may soon be a moot point for nurses prepared at the graduate level, because no one denies that the nurse practitioner role involves cure work.

So far, then, we have looked at two arenas of nursing as cure work: the domains of chronic care and primary practice. In chronic care, admitting that nurses do cure work is simply a new perspective on an old role. For the most part, the nurse is doing tasks she has always done. In some cases—in certain kinds of patient teaching, for example—she is doing work she was taught how to do but possibly prohibited from doing because of physician dominance and control.

In primary care, the nurse has acquired a new set of skills. Here, the nurse does what the physician would do, were he present. Granted, she may do it better because of her simultaneous sensitivity to care needs, but the research shows that she does it with skill equal to the physician's.

For simplicity, we will label theories about these two sorts of cure as substitution theories because the nurse generally substitutes for the physician. But these cure philosophies are only the tip of the iceberg.

CURE: THE NEW CONCEPTS

Not all nurses who advocate cure see it as a substitution for medicine. Interesting new patterns have crept into the so-called cure work. Watson (1979) apparently has made the traditional differentiation between care and cure in deriving her so-called carative factors: "The term carative is used to contrast to the more common term

curative to help the student to differentiate nursing and medicine."
(p. 7)

On further inspection, however, one can see that she has shifted
the traditional meanings of care and cure: "Whereas curative factors
aim at curing the patient of disease, carative factors aim at the caring
process that helps the person attain (or maintain) health or die a
peaceful death." (Watson, 1979, p. 7)

In this formulation, Watson has associated curing with disease
in its most narrow meaning. On the other hand, she has associated
caring with healing the person. In that way, although eschewing
curing for nurses, she has brought them into the activity of healing.
In effect, this formulation has brought nursing into the commonsense
notion of curing, or, one might say, has made *curing* a limited aspect
of a larger concept, *healing*. Caring, according to Watson, is more
"healthogenic" than is curing (p. 9).

A similar difference between healing and curing has been made
by McGlone (1990), who noted that a disease is cured, whereas a
person is healed. For McGlone, healing means to be made whole, an
awakening of a deeper sense of self (p. 78).

Quinn (1989) also described healing as the realm of the nurse.
However, Quinn views the nurse not so much as healer but as midwife
to an internal process in the patient:

> *Healing is a total, organismic, synergistic response that must emerge
> from within the individual if recovery and growth are to be accom-
> plished. . . . The Haelan Effect is the activation of the innate, diverse,
> synergistic, and multidimensional self-healing mechanism which mani-
> fests as emergence and repatterning of relationship (p. 554).*

Although Watson described the nurse's role more strongly, she
has not always been consistent in her use of terms and, in at least
one book (Watson, 1988a), advocated synthesizing care and cure. As
she stated, "Care is not proposed as simply a secondary fall-back
position when cure is impossible. . . . Caring then becomes the
ethical principle or standard by which (curing) interventions are
measured." (p. 2)

Notice the change in tactics. In 1979, Watson left cure to physicians but narrowed its application. Here, she subordinated it to care.

Leininger (1991) used the strategy of subordinating cure to care:
"Care (caring) is essential to curing and healing, for there can be no
curing without caring." (p. 45)

Watson and Leininger both enhanced nursing's domain but decreased medicine's, sometimes by manipulating the meaning of the
terms *caring* and *curing* (Watson, 1979) and sometimes by asserting
the dominance of care over cure (Watson, 1988a; Leininger, 1991).

Both Leininger and Watson linked their wide-spectrum care constructs to unique contexts. For Leininger, the context is cultural; for Watson, it is a world characterized by aspects associated with the emerging new world paradigm. One may get a quick flavor of Watson's (1998b) context from the following quotations:

> A person's body is confined in time and space, but the mind and soul are not confined to the physical universe. One's higher sense of mind and soul transcends time and space and helps to account for notions like collective unconscious, causal past, mystical experiences, parapsychological phenomena, a higher sense of power, and may be an indicator of the spiritual evolution of human beings (p. 50).
>
> The concept of the soul, as used here refers to the geist, spirit, inner self, or essence of the person, which is tied to a greater sense of self-awareness, a higher degree of consciousness, an inner strength, and a power that can expand human capacities and allow a person to transcend his or her usual self. The higher sense of consciousness and valuing of inner-self can cultivate a fuller access to the intuitive and even sometimes allow uncanny, mystical, or miraculous experiences....
>
> One's ability to transcend space and time occurs in a similar manner through one's mind, imagination, and emotions. Our bodies may be physically present in a given location or situation, but our minds and related feelings may be located elsewhere (p. 46).

By characterizing her world in this way, Watson chose New Age ideologies and an alternate healing modality. Watson's nurse enters cure work because cure is no longer associated with the body, but with the individual's evolving and developing personhood. The perception of disease has changed; as Watson has said, it results from disharmony in the person. If the nurse is instrumental, then, in restoring harmony, she is involved in cure work.

Interestingly, the term *curing* is more often associated with the traditional medical model (and its related world view), whereas the term *healing* is typically associated with the newly emerging paradigm. Although there certainly is crossover in use of these terms, curing and healing tend to evoke different images. Although Watson used the term *curing*, her connotations frequently evoke the notion of healing instead.

NONNURSING HEALING MOVEMENTS

It is interesting to compare Watson's ideology and the education offered to her students with the ideology and practices of one of the newer healing programs. Watson's material lends itself to the comparison because of the similar world context. The Barbara Brennan School of Healing is used for this comparison. Brennan's (1987) world is reminiscent of Watson's:

> *There is abundant evidence that many human beings today are expand-*
> *ing the usual five senses into super-sensory levels. Most people have*
> *High Sense Perception to some degree, without necessarily realizing*
> *it. . . . It is possible that there is already a transformation in conscious-*
> *ness taking place and that more people are developing a new sense*
> *in which information is received on a different and possibly higher*
> *frequency (pp. 9–10).*

Brennan, who is not a nurse, holds a graduate degree in physics. Probably for that reason, she is more definitive in describing her alternate world view than is Watson, but one suspects Watson would have little difficulty understanding Brennan's "dynamic web of inseparable energy patterns," her notion of holistic awareness, and her assertion that "holistic awareness will be outside linear time and three-dimensional space and therefore will not be easily recognized. We must practice holistic experience to be able to recognize it." (Brennan, 1987, p. 26) The world of holistic experience that Brennan's students are taught to use for healing involves High Sense Perception of patients' and their human conditions. For visualizers, this may include seeing the patients' auras and chakras (described as perceptible to those who have developed the ability to see at higher levels of vibration). Other students may, instead, have High Sense Perception through other senses, for example, touch.

Brennan's context is one in which multiple worlds exist in the same space, vibrating at different levels, making them, not unlike radio waves, undetectable except to those who can alter their vibratory rates of perception. Brennan's students use their hands to work in these altered frequencies, manipulating a patient's energy—pushing, pulling, or stopping it—to produce healing.

Watson's theory seems vulnerable to criticism when it assumes that all nurses will be caring—despite Watson's admission that varying degrees of the trait exist. There is no great assurance that her theory would eliminate the "bad apples" (those without affective caring for their patients). Keep in mind that this criticism does not refer to the weeding out of such students in the given program at the University of Colorado; it deals with the question of whether Watson's theory *itself* provides for that contingency. And it is difficult to say that it does.

Brennan's healing program, on the other hand, has built-in controls, some pragmatic, some conceptual. First, her students are required to be in personal therapy. In essence, they are required to do the personal growth that Watson's theory talks about but does not seem to guarantee.

More important, Brennan's program deals directly with the High Sense Perception of students. A major focus of the program is on clarifying the reception. Interpreting perceptions from higher vibrational levels *accurately* happens as a matter of both training and personal growth and development. And these elements compose a major part of Brennan's theory as well as her program. A fallback position of this sort would enhance Watson's theory, were it possible.

Brennan's healing philosophy handles flaws of body and psyche with the same therapies, treating the person as if from whole cloth. Furthermore, Brennan's healing therapies often are used simultaneously with modern medicine. Because they treat different phenomena (energy bodies and human bodies, respectively), there is no perceived conflict, even though both modalities share the goal of healing. The inherent interplay of body and psyche in Brennan's theory reminds one of Watson's assertion that disease arises from disharmony.

Some readers may be disturbed by these atypical notions of reality; but in studying theory, it is essential to put aside such reactions. In Chapter 13, we will see that there are two aspects to theory analysis. Internal criticism looks for consistency and coherency of the theory's components as they intersect. External criticism then asks the question, Yes, but does the theory reflect the real world?

One should not allow a negative answer to the second question to prevent a reasoned internal critique. In essence, the question for internal analysis is, If one were to accept as a given the worlds described by Brennan and Watson, how consistent are their theories with their proposed world views? I am suggesting that Brennan's theory is adequate to deal with her subject matter and Watson's may have a few gaps.

One could argue whether Brennan's advantage was gained because of a more coherent theory or whether the subject matter of healing *fits* more easily into the new paradigm than does the more ambiguous topic of nursing. Is Watson doing something interesting but not what all would call *nursing*? More about internal and external criticism later.

In terms of the notion of therapeutic touch itself, the use of touch in the typical nursing model and the Brennan model are far apart, namely in the degree of skill required and the level of personal development needed by the healer. Although Krieger (1981) has admitted that there are levels of expertise in therapeutic touch, her claim is that, "basically, Therapeutic Touch is an act which nurses engage in quite naturally in the course of their nursing practice" (p.

138). On a primitive level, therapeutic touch is an instinctive act. Therapeutic touch, as promulgated in nursing, often is conveyed as a learned psychomotor skill, simply a technique for moving the hands over the patient's body and sensing changes in the patient's energy field. The technique can be taught to any interested nurse in a few days or a few hours in a concentrated workshop, so say some teachers in these programs. Often the nurses are told of associated elements of centering and intention, but few workshops attempt to test for achievement of these states.

Keegan (1989) has described the four phases of therapeutic touch as follows:

1. centering oneself physically and psychologically; this is finding within oneself an inner reference of stability
2. exercising the natural sensitivity of the hand to assess the energy field of the client for clues to differentiate the quality of energy flow
3. mobilizing areas in the client's energy field that the healer may perceive as being nonflowing, that is, sluggish, congested, or static
4. the conscious direction by the healer of his or her excess body energies to assist the client to repattern his or her own energies (p. 258).

Notice there is no direct reference to the nature of the healer herself. Or as Heidt (1990) has said, "The nurse's field of energy may be characterized as being 'well' or 'whole'; the patient's energy field, as 'less whole.'" (p. 180)

Brennan, I suspect, would call this an untested assumption. In contrast to the nursing model (that generally assumes all nurses qualify), Brennan has a 4-year program in which the healer's personal growth and her skills in directing energy through her hands are simultaneously developed and verified.

For Brennan, there are levels of perception, and the ability to manipulate energy at those various levels depends on the learner's own evolution. The student's growth and psychic development allow her to develop and refine her High Sense Perception, using this sense to discern different levels of the patient's being, each level finer (at a higher vibration level) than the level beneath it. Only when these levels are perceived through one or more of the senses can the healer work with them with full clarity and understanding of what she is doing.

Do nurse teachers of therapeutic touch require any sort of high sense perception on the part of those learning the skill? Do they have methods of validating the student's skill—namely serious and independent testing to see if an instructor and a student are perceiving the same energy patterns (a critical part of Brennan's education)?

I hope there are nursing groups that have such safeguards, but, if so, they are exceptions. The only validation in many nursing teaching programs involves the mere confirmation by the student that she "feels" the energy (patients make similar confirmations). Seldom is there any attempt to see if the student and instructor "feel" the same thing.

In essence, the popular nursing concept of therapeutic touch is that it is a technique of moving the hands, a technique any willing nurse can learn, a technique not unlike starting an intravenous line. The right movements, a bit of sensitivity to radiating energies, and anyone can do it.

For Brennan, healing touch is a skill that develops as the healer develops, not a simplistic technique to be exercised by anyone. Brennan would grant that some untrained people have the ability, but she would not grant that the mechanical moving of hands over a patient's body—without the appropriate mental preparation, without knowledgeable control of energies through them—could be effective except in a serendipitous accidental fashion.

Essentially, the issues here are two-fold: (1) whether the act of touch can be systematically effective apart from extensive training with verification and (2) whether the healer herself must have attained certain levels of personal development and requisite certain states of mind in which to exercise the skill.

The rapid growth of healing phenomena is one of the more interesting facets of the so-called New Age world view. Although nurses have been heavily involved in healing and healing therapies, the territory of healing has not been claimed by the nursing profession—nor is it likely to be. Many of the most successful healers are not nurses, and the therapies associated with healing are not taught in most nursing programs.

Of course, many of the nurses who move into healing work come from programs like Watson's, curricula that stress holistic theories, often those more or less linked to Martha Rogers's (1970) theory. Although not all holistic theories embrace healing, many have a context not unlike that proposed by Watson or Brennan.

The holistic nursing movement (in many of its formulations) grants that nurses may be agents of cure. If the therapies advanced are associated with cure (like therapeutic touch), then the theory sees cure work as belonging in nursing.

Unlike the cure theories advanced by Loomis and Wood and unlike the cure work of nurse practitioners, holistic theories typically offer cure work that little resembles the cure work of physicians.

Cure is the goal, but the therapies are radically different. Almost invariably, these theories are grounded in an alternate world paradigm.

SUMMARY

The issue of care versus cure is more complex than it might appear at first glance. There is the basic question of whether health care actions can truly be segregated on this basis. Is every act of a health care worker aimed specifically at either care or cure? Can the same act serve both goals? Can the same act serve one goal at one time and its supposed opposite at another?

Must the content of medicine and nursing remain inviolable? Border-setting between nursing and medicine can be seen as a political decision rather than an eternal truth. The difference may be what we chose to make it in our particular nation at a particular time in history.

Indeed, one might contrast the system in the United States with that in the various Russian countries. In their system, the nursing function is structured as an interim rung on the way to medicine. In that system, the two professions are not differentiated in kind but are joined on a continuum.

When the difference between the two professions is interpreted as a matter of policy rather than of fact, there are at least two critical boundary events. The first is the resolutions at law; the second is the ongoing changes in social behaviors. In relation to the first, nursing is what the laws of a state say it is. At present, in every state in the United States, a physician may legally practice nursing, but a nurse may not legally practice medicine.

And always, changes in practice precede changes at law: *de facto* then *de jure*. In this country, that means nurses at the cutting edge are always vulnerable to being charged with exceeding the privileges of their licenses.

Caring and curing are perennial goals in health care. The relationship of nursing to and with these goals has fluctuated over the centuries. At present, there are numerous movements to account for both of these goals within the scope of nursing practice. Nevertheless, a large number of nurses and nurse theorists still use care versus cure as the demarcation between the professions of nursing and medicine.

In addition, it is impossible to say out of context what either term (*caring* or *curing*) means. Nursing theorists have given both terms many and varied shifts in connotation and denotation. When reading a work of theory concerning care or cure, it is particularly important to discern how the author uses these terms.

REFERENCES

Brennan, B. A. (1987). *Hands of light: A guide to healing through the human energy field*. New York: Bantam Books.
Hall, L. E. (1968). Another view of nursing care and quality. *Maryland Nursing News, 1*, 1–5.
Heidt, P. R. (1990). Openness: A qualitative analysis of nurses' and patients' experiences of therapeutic touch. *Image, 3*, 180–186.
Keegan, L. (1989). Touch: Connecting with the healing power. In B. M. Dossey, L. Keegan, L. G. Kolkmeirer, & C. E. Guzetta, *Holistic health promotion: A guide for practice* (pp. 249–272). Rockville, MD: Aspen Publishers.
Krieger, D. (1981). *Foundations for holistic health nursing practices: The renaissance nurse*. Philadelphia: J.B. Lippincott.
Leininger, M. M. (1991). The theory of culture care diversity and universality. In M. M. Leininger (Ed.), *Culture care diversity & universality: A theory of nursing* (pp. 5–68). New York: National League for Nursing.
Loomis, M. E., & Wood, D. J. (1983). Cure: The potential outcome of nursing care. *Image, 1*, 4–7.
McGlone, M. E. (1990). Healing the spirit. *Holistic Nursing Practice, 4*, 77–84.
Quinn, J. F. (1989). On healing, wholeness, and the Haelan Effect. *Nursing & Health Care, 10*, 552–556.
Rogers, M. E. (1970). *An introduction to the theoretical basis of nursing*. Philadelphia: F. A. Davis.
Watson, J. (1979). *Nursing: The philosophy and science of caring*. Boston: Little, Brown.
Watson, J. (1988a). Introduction: An ethic of caring/curing/nursing qua nursing. In J. Watson & M. A. Ray (Eds.), *The ethics of care and the ethics of cure: Synthesis in chronicity* (pp. 1–3). New York: National League for Nursing.
Watson, J. (1988b). *Nursing: Human science and human care: A theory of nursing*. New York: National League for Nursing.

BIBLIOGRAPHY

Geary, P. A., & Hawkins, J. W. (1991). To cure, to care, or to heal. *Nursing Forum, 3*, 5–13.
Kinlein, M. L. (1977). *Independent nursing practice with clients*. Philadelphia: J.B. Lippincott.
Krieger, D. (1979). *The therapeutic touch: How to use your hands to help or to heal*. Englewood Cliffs, NJ: Prentice-Hall.
MacNutt, F. (1977). *The power to heal*. Notre Dame, IN: Ave Maria Press.
Oliver, N. R. (1990). Nurse are you a healer? *Nursing Forum, 2*, 11–14.
Quinn, J. F. (1992). Holding sacred space: The nurse as healing environment. *Holistic Nursing Practice, 4*, 26–36.
Reed, P. G. (1990). Toward a nursing theory of self-transcendence: Deductive reformulation using developmental theories. *Advances in Nursing Science, 1*, 64–77.

8   *Holistic Nursing Theories*

Holistic theories represent the fastest growing trend in nursing. A *holistic theory* is one whose subject matter is conceptualized as an indivisible whole, an entity that is fractured and distorted if considered as a collection of parts. Most often the subject matter of holistic theories is man, but some holistic theories take the universe or health as subject matter. Whatever their subject matter, holistic theories share a commitment not to see their subject matter as an accumulation of parts. This means that they take a view counter to the predominant medical model as well as to many popular nursing models.

THE INFLUENCE OF ROGERS

Martha Rogers (1970, 1990) was one of the earlier nurse theorists to promulgate a holistic theory. Indeed, many subsequent theorists have adopted her holistic notions of man and environment. As she said,

> The unity of man is a reality. Man interacts with his environment in his totality. Only as man's wholeness is perceived does the study of man begin to yield meaningful concepts and theories. Only as man's oneness is apprehended is it possible to identify man's distinctive attributes (Rogers, 1970. p. 44).
>
> Nursing is the study of unitary, irreducible, indivisible human and environmental fields: people and their world. . . . [P]eople are energy fields. They do not have them. All reality is postulated to be multidimensional as defined herein. One does not become multidimensional. Rather, this is a way of perceiving reality (Rogers, 1990, pp. 5–6).

Rogers's original theory focused around four principles: (1) *reciprocy* (interaction between human and environmental fields); (2) *synchrony* (a function of the human/environmental field interacting at a point in space–time); (3) *helicy* (subsuming reciprocy and

Barbara J. Stevens Barnum: NURSING THEORY:
ANALYSIS, APPLICATION, EVALUATION, FOURTH EDITION.
© 1994, 1990, 1984, 1979 J.B. Lippincott.

synchrony and describing the unidirectional life process as characterized by probabilistic goal directedness); and (4) *resonancy* (purporting that change in pattern and organization of the human and environmental field is propagated in waves; Rogers, 1970, pp. 95–103).

Her newer version has reduced those principles to three:

1. Principle of resonancy: Continuous change from lower to
   higher frequency wave patterns in human and environmental
   fields
2. Principle of helicy: Continuous innovative, unpredictable,
   increasing diversity of human and environmental field
   patterns
3. Principle of integrality: Continuous mutual human field and
   environmental field process (Rogers, 1990, p. 8).

Although these principles may seem complex, especially because
Rogers has created her own vocabulary, a close examination reveals
a world paradigm not unlike that of Watson and Brennan.

THEORISTS IN THE ROGERIAN TRADITION

Newman, Parse, Fitzpatrick, and many other holistic nurse theorists
have credited Rogers with having been the inspiration for their work.
Rogers's (1970) early book, known as the "Purple Book" by her students, primarily portrayed a view of the world and man. There was
much room for students to take her world view and expand on it or
to evolve specifics of nursing therapy compatible with her view.

Take, for example, the work of Black and Haight (1992), who
applied Rogers's principle of integrality to late-life development.
They looked at the final phase of life review through the principle
of integrality, and differentiated between mere reminiscing and an
integrality that included evaluating and garnering insight from the
life experience (pp. 8–9).

Today, there are many nurses with holistic theories who believe
they are doing "the same thing" because of their mutual beginnings
in Rogers's work. In fact, once you look at the theories (e.g., those
of Newman [1979, 1986], Parse [1981], and Krieger [1979, 1981]), it
is clear that each has added unique components and taken slightly
different directions.

Sometimes the differences among holistic theories have to do
with focus rather then substance. For example, some of these theories
look more closely at health than at man, and some take the opposite
course. The reader may get a taste of holistic theory differences and
similarities from the representative citations given in this chapter.

Newman (1986) virtually joined the subjects of health and man by saying that the natural evolution of man *is* health. For Newman, health is equated with the evolution of consciousness. Like Watson, she has followed closely the models of psychology cited in the transpersonal literature:

> *The process of the evolution of consciousness is also the process of health. The human being comes from a state of potential consciousness into the world of determinate matter and has the capacity for understanding that will enable him or her to gain insight regarding his/her pattern. This instantaneous insight represents a turning point in evolving consciousness with concomitant gains in freedom (p. 43).*
>
> *. . . the "flow of life" [is] seen as a kaleidoscopic evolution of patterning with paradoxes, contradictions, and ambiguities continually being synthesized into insights that lead to an ever-expanding consciousness. The revolutional [sic] conceptualization of Newman's paradigm is the proposition that health is the synthesis of disease/nondisease. Newman's model embraces a dialectical outlook where transformation is basic, where the fundamental unit of analysis is movement, and where disease and nondisease are each reflections of a larger whole (p. 111).*

The focus on patterning is reminiscent of Rogers's (1970) early work, where she said such things as "Pattern and organization have become basic concepts in contemporary efforts to achieve a better understanding of human growth and behavior" (p. 61) or "The life process possesses its own dynamic pattern and organization. The patterning that takes place over time is evolutionary in nature and encompasses the unity of life." (p. 62)

Newman (1986) also has adopted Rogers's notion of energy fields:

> *Although we cannot always "see" energy exchange, we accept that it is a characteristic of the human field (e.g. the energy patterns depicted by a electrocardiogram or electroencephalogram). Disease makes it possible for us to envision a total pattern of the energy field of a person. For example, hypertension may connote a pattern of contained energy, hyperthyroidism a pattern of diffuse, multidirectional energy, or diabetes the inability to use available energy (pp. 22–23).*

Krieger (1981), following Rogers's work, took a holistic perspective of health in which man and environment are both essential components:

> *The underlying premise of holistic health practices is that it is a major misconception of our times that the germ theory accounts for all illness. . . . This means that illness is the product of a complementary interaction between mind and body under conditions of stress that*

cannot be reconciled. The goal of the holistic perspective is to treat all aspects of the person's problems by an integrated approach that consid-ers both the person in the context of the problem and the problem in the context of the uniqueness of the individual, thus giving the situation a more humanistic orientation than has previously been the case (pp. 79–80).

Parse (1981), like Rogers, developed her own vocabulary of pre-ferred terms. The following is a discussion of what she called the "coconstituting" of man and environment:

Assumption 1 synthesized the concepts of coexistence, coconstitution, and pattern and organization. The assumption means that man exists with others, evolving simultaneously and in cadence with the environ-ment. Man, a recognizable pattern in the man–environment interrela-tionship, unfolds with contemporaries the ideas of predecessors. This interrelationship is the continuity that connects past with future, bearing witness to man's coexistence with all men. . . .

Man and environment, then, interchange energy to create what is in the world, and man chooses the meaning given to the situations he cocreates. Man is responsible for all outcomes of choices even though he does not know them when making a decision (pp. 26–27).

In essence, most holistic theories in nursing take a transcendental view of man or reality, that is, they perceive the most real facets of existence to be principles and experiences that reach beyond the concrete, measurable, everyday experience. Furthermore, they share a general displeasure with any reductionist thinking, that is, with any theory that explains a thing by reference to its parts.

NON-ROGERIAN HOLISM

Not all holistic theories lend evidence that they were direct spin-offs from Rogers. Kolcaba (1992), for example, devised a map for holistic comfort that would be compatible with a more traditional world view, yet still preserved the holism. Her model is designed to create, as she has said, a nurse-sensitive outcome (p. 1). In her grid, she interfaced two sets of variables so that comfort would be seen as a multidimensional personal experience, with different degrees of intensity. Her cognitive map looks at physical, psychospiritual, environmental, and social factors as they cross-grid against states of relief, ease, or transcendence.

Selder (1989) also developed a holistic theory that was neither derived from nor representative of Rogers's unitary man paradigm. Hers is a theory of life transition, described as follows:

> *A life transition is initiated when a person's current reality is disrupted.*
> *The disruption of the reality can originate in a crucial event or from a*
> *determined decision. . . .*
>   *Life transition theory describes how people restructure their reality*
> *and resolve uncertainty, a major characteristic of any transition. The*
> *shape of the transition is the resolution of the uncertainty (p. 437).*

Although Selder's (1989) theory retains a holistic approach to man, it focuses on the unique perceptions of the person undergoing transition. For example, in relation to the perception of time (one of the elements altered by transition), she said,

> *During the life transition there are changes in the perception of time.*
> *Following a disruption in reality, the person's sense of time is collapsed;*
> *there is no orientation to the future as far as time is concerned, there*
> *is preoccupation with the predisrupted reality (p. 451).*

Selder's model is middle range, that is, not purporting to apply to all persons or even all persons labeled as patients. It applies to a single class: those who have experienced a major life disruption. Her own work has involved many patients who fit in this category, for example, patients suffering spinal cord injuries.

Fitzpatrick (1983) also is concerned with temporal patterns, but extended her theory to all mankind:

> *This life perspective rhythm model . . . proposes that the process of*
> *human development is characterized by rhythms. . . . Throughout the*
> *developmental process one can identify peaks and troughs of particular*
> *human rhythms with the overall progression toward faster rhythms. For*
> *example, in relation to temporal patterns one can identify the basic*
> *progression of the rhythm as moving from time passing slowly, through*
> *time passing quickly, toward timelessness (p. 300).*

It is easy to see that these two theories (Selder and Fitzpatrick) could be compatible if filtered through the same view; yet the Selder theory could be valid in a more traditional view as well. Not all holistic theories have to view the world through the same paradigm. The fact that many holistic theories come out of Rogerian notions or New Age ideology is happenstance, not necessity. And some theories—like Selder's—might apply in more than one construct.

HOLISTIC THEORIES: WEAKNESSES AND STRENGTHS

Man in his totality is the subject matter for most holistic theories of nursing. Some theorists, like Newman, have equated health with human development; others like Watson, have viewed health as a form of human harmony. Holistic theories face a boundary problem when it comes to nursing, and we could rightly ask, How does the nurse differ from the transpersonal psychologist? Often these theories are dense with world context, heavy on how man is seen in his environment, and thin on what nurses actually do. In other cases, there is a strange dichotomy between what nurses do in their practice and the topics that the theories discuss.

Another problem related to these theories can be asked this way: If nursing is the study of man in his totality, how does that relate to the fact that nursing is usually seen as a practical art? More specifically, the average man thinks of a nurse as someone who helps when his health fails. If many of these holistic theories are to be taken literally, there is no more justification for a nurse when someone is ill than when that person is well. It seems that everyone needs a nurse (someone to assist in their human development) apart from considerations of wellness or illness. And, if that is so, how can a person be convinced that the nurse has the knowledge and skills necessary to be that lifetime guide?

In taking a holistic image of man as its subject matter, nursing is able to contrast its subject matter (whole man) with medicine's (man as his physiologic body systems, man as a collection of diseases). The common assertion of holistic nursing theories is that medicine treats the disease, whereas nursing treats the person. This is not to say that physicians would agree with this interpretation.

THE QUESTION OF METHOD IN HOLISM

Another issue raised by holistic theories is how one studies, researches, or even practices within a whole that cannot be divided. Some theorists get around this problem by having the nurse "intuit" the patient, somewhat akin to the old philosophic argument given by Gibson (1960) in relation to social enquiry:

> The central notion, as we have seen, is that we understand what is going on simply by participating in it. This is easily recognized in the case of ourselves; we live through our own experiences, and in doing so become aware of them. But we also participate, along with others, in social processes, and in doing this are able to grasp the situation not only from our own point of view, but from theirs. By identifying ourselves with them, we come to feel what they feel, or at any rate to think their thoughts (p. 50).

Others have not had a problem separating out aspects of the whole on a temporary provisional basis. Krieger (1981) described the mechanism this way:

> In terms of humans, the plan of the whole means that practices to support a person's health must keep the self-identity of the "whole" person in mind and must recognize that it is from this enduring perspective that each individual perceives intrinsic reality. This intrinsic reality, based as it is upon the individual's life history, in turn lends the individual personality a unity of character for its expression. Consequently, the emerging stance of the holistic health practitioner is to strive to understand simultaneously the relationship of the "part" of the individual under concern to the totality of that individual's interactions and the relationship of the whole to its parts (p. 4).

Moccia (1986) also addressed the topic of how one considers parts in a holistic theory:

> Once holism is assumed, one must find a way to recognize, acknowledge, respect and account for the inevitable distortions that occur when the indivisible totality is artificially divided, as is necessary. Such a process is described within a dialectical understanding of reality by the act of individuation, which is "simply a matter of carving up the whole in a different manner for a particular purpose." I have argued elsewhere that this concept offers nursing scholarship a way out of the theoretical paradox that comes with holism (p. 31).

Newman (1986) may be on thinner ice when she accepted use of a tool specifically associated with a reductionist theory:

> In spite of this belief that pattern recognition is more a matter of being able to "read" one's own pattern than of collecting information "external" to oneself, an assessment framework may be useful in initial efforts to identify pattern. The assessment framework developed by the nurse theorist group of the North American Nursing Diagnosis Association (NANDA) is consistent with the paradigm of health presented here (p. 73).

Although one may quibble concerning which methods have infringed too sharply on the indivisible whole, it is clear that one can look at the same subject matter through various colored glasses (i.e., partialities) as a method of individuating and yet preserving the whole. To look at Levine's (1971) theory in a holistic fashion, for example, one might look at the whole patient through energy-colored glasses at one time and structure-colored glasses at another without destroying the integrity and unity of the whole man.

Holistic theories have both a philosophic value (a commitment not to see things in a reductionist fashion) and an obligation to find appropriate practice/research/learning methods. Because the classical experimental design, with its manipulation of variables, breaks things into components, it is difficult to combine with holism. Holism has found more acceptable methods in qualitative research involving phenomenology or hermeneutics. Both of these methods involve exploring the lived experience as it is immediately experienced; both aim for a deeper understanding of the phenomenon observed, with hermeneutics focusing on the interpretation of such experience.

Because these methods are favored, it is common to find holistic theorists interested in conditions of the human soul or spirit—or the emotive aspects of experience that arise concurrently with illness of any sort. For example, Dugan (1989) analyzed sadness, fear, and anger, finding that these human conditions can, if prolonged and deep, develop into states of illness: depression, anxiety, and hostility/ resentment respectively.

Globally, then, one could say theorists who are reductionists (focus on the parts) tend to use quantitative research and classical experimental design. Advocates of holistic theories, on the other hand, usually prefer qualitative research. Because the two philosophies represent different ways of viewing the world (in wholes, in parts), it is not surprising that they differ as to what sources will be taken as valid in searching for truth. Benner (1985) has stated the problem from the perspective of qualitative research:

> The paradox of the subject/object split of Cartesian dualism is that it is either extremely subjectivizing or extremely objectifying. The self is viewed as a possession and attributes are given objectively as possessions by the subject in a purely intentional way. This view cannot take account of the historical, cultural, embodied, situated person (p. 2).

Some researchers simply cannot accept methods that fail to objectify and isolate variables. They insist that qualitative research cannot lead to knowledge. Researchers who favor qualitative research (and that includes most who adopt holistic theories) believe that much of what is significant is lost in the very act of objectifying and isolating parts. Of course, not every researcher is for one method and against the other. Nurses increasingly are coming to realize that each method has much to offer. But phenomenology and hermeneutics fit well with holistic theory development because they allow for the study of a subject matter in its entirety, without artificially separating it into pieces.

One may look behind the reductionist and holistic methods of research and find that they represent different methods of thinking. To use the nursing process, for example, the nurse must divide things into steps and pieces in her mind, calling forth thought patterns that look at the parts. In contrast, the dialectic thought process, which moves by striving to blend perceived components into larger, more comprehensive wholes, allows for holism. The approach is compatible with phenomenology, yet can be separated from it.

There are an increasing number of holistic theories of nursing, particularly because phenomenology and hermeneutics have gained respect in the profession as methods of research. There is also an increased use of dialectic reasoning.

Because most nurses are counseled to treat the whole patient, not the incision, not the broken leg, holistic philosophies appeal to many. Indeed, these theories are threatening to eclipse the nursing process in popularity.

A holistic approach must be differentiated from a comprehensive one. Many theorists have mistakenly claimed to be holistic when they actually meant that they considered all the parts. Considering all the pieces is *not* a holistic tactic. A holistic phenomenon has only one essence in which all aspects participate. The two notions of wholeness are antithetical ways of viewing man and the world.

HOLISTIC CURING

In Chapter 7, we said that the holistic nursing movement often advocates the nurse as cure agent. Indeed, many practitioners of holistic nursing claim they have created viable cure alternatives to medical practice, Others claim they do curing work that is compatible with and even complementary to medicine.

Holistic nurse practitioners often adopt independent nursing interventions that may be applied with a curing, rather than a caring, intention (or they may be applied as both anodyne and cure simultaneously). Therapeutic touch (Krieger, 1981; Quinn, 1988) was the first such method to gain extensive popularity, although it has been followed by others. As Krieger (1981) said about therapeutic touch,

> *Therapeutic Touch derives from, but is not the same as, the ancient art of the laying-on of hands. The major points of difference between Therapeutic Touch and the laying-on of hands are methodological; Therapeutic Touch has no religious base as does the laying-on-of hands; it is a conscious, intentional act; it is based on research findings; and Therapeutic Touch does not require a declaration of faith from the healee (patient) for it to be effective (p. 138).*

Therapeutic touch is not always separated from a religious aspect or spiritual aspect as we will see in Chapter 9, although where the two aspects are conjoined often the spiritual interpretation is closer to New Age beliefs than to older religious forms.

Krieger, like many holistic theorists, has mixed caring and curing without worrying about their boundaries. It is clear, however, that her use of the term *healer* is not to be taken lightly. For Krieger, cure is within the scope of her practice. Therapeutic touch has remained one of the chief methods used in holistic curing. As mentioned in Chapter 7, nonnurse healers also place much stress on therapeutic use of the hands, though technique and understanding of what is happening may vary.

Barrett (1990) has given generic descriptions of methods that she sees as developing under the holistic theory of Rogers. She raised the point that human contact may be an important part of the procedures:

> *Practice modalities are options that can be used by clients to pursue a way of living, to assist in lifestyle change, to increase awareness of opportunities to be well, and to provide information that may be helpful in making health-related choices.*
>
> *Many modalities can promote power enhancement whereby clients use their capacity to participate knowingly in change to actualize certain potentials....*
>
> *At times the deliberative mutual patterning process itself is the healing modality. This is the case when human therapeutic contact is deemed essential to enhancing the health of the person* (p. 34).

New holistic methods are numerous, and a wide armamentarium of techniques is developing rapidly. Hare (1988), for example, has explored shiatsu acupressure, a method akin to acupuncture, and Titlebaum (1988) has discussed relaxation therapy. Ruxton (1988) and Dugan (1989), following Norman Cousins's (1979) lead, have explored humor in its curative potential. Barnum (1989) has discussed the lending of energy and White (1988) has expanded on the use of the hands for therapeutic massage. Zahourek (1987) has explored clinical hypnosis and Brallier (1988) has used biofeedback. Guzzetta (1989) has added music therapy to the list and Barbara M. Dossey (1989a) has worked with centering.

It is often difficult to categorize these methods as care work or cure work. For example, Kist (1992) has used acupuncture to keep pregnant drug abusers clean in the latter months of pregnancy. How could this successful therapy be classified as care or cure?

Vines (1988), Krieger (1981), and B. Dossey (1989b) all have used guided imagery, possibly the second most popular technique after therapeutic touch. B. Dossey (1989b) described guided imagery this way: "The goal of the imagery process is for a person to create an *end-result* image of reaching one's potential that directly evokes positive psychophysiologic responses." (p. 159)

B. Dossey's (1989c) explanation for the effectiveness of imagery is as follows:

> *None of the body systems is separate from the other, for images and stressors perceived by the person's mind are transduced to the messenger*

molecules—the neurotransmitters of the autonomic nervous system and the hormones of the endocrine system. Recent evidence from PNI [psychoneuroimmunology] researchers shows that there is a bidirectional information circuitry operating between the immune system and the autonomic and endocrine systems (p. 61).

Vines (1988) has concurred with B. Dossey, noting that mental images are not pictures in the mind but notions that may be integrated with the individual's physiologic response patterns (p. 36).

Like therapeutic touch, these alternate interventions have been adopted by nurses more often than by physicians. The notions involved in these holistic practices cut against the grain of the dominant medical theory, although inroads have been made among the physician population by new paradigm works such as those by physician Larry Dossey (1982).

Holistic methods may appeal to the nurse for several reasons. For one, the methods are there for the begging, because most physicians still want little to do with them. In addition, the notion of human response on levels other than anatomical structure and physiologic function is appealing to the nurse who has been educated to view the patient as a whole. As B. Dossey (1989c) has explained, though, such methods may have more of a anatomic/physiologic base than is usually credited to them. In any case, holistic methods offer the possibility of avoiding the reductionism that is the crux of the holistic complaint against other nursing theories.

Holism, then, whether applied to the patient, to health, or to the whole of reality, is a commitment to seeing the subject matter as indivisible, not as a composition of smaller parts. Holism is not a method but a philosophy, a commitment to viewing a thing in its entirety. It is most compatible with a phenomenologic approach to research and a dialectic thought process. Both of these elements are discussed later in this book.

SUMMARY

Most present holistic theories of nursing deal with interesting, emerging content such as transpersonal psychology, aspects of transition and temporality, and concepts of self-growth as cure. Inherently fascinating, these subjects must be analyzed carefully in order to evaluate whether they represent the appropriate domain for a profession of nursing. Not every nurse will reach the same conclusion.

The holistic theories tend to be presented within a New Age ideology, though some few are contained in or compatible with a traditional world view. Subject matters of these theories range from man to health to human evolution to the universe itself.

At present holistic theories vie for predominance with those based on nursing process or nursing diagnosis. These two sorts of theory form a new professional dichotomy, one that holds little hope for resolution. Will the two philosophies, with their related methods, develop two radically different schools and tracks of nursing education? Or will one side eventually become normative? It is an interesting era, and the answer is yet to be determined.

REFERENCES

Barnum, B. J. (1989). Expanded consciousness: Nurses' experiences. *Nursing Outlook, 6*, 260–266.

Barrett, E.A.M. (1990). Rogers' science-based nursing practice. In E.A.M. Barrett (Ed.), *Visions of Rogers' science-based nursing* (pp. 31–44). New York: National League for Nursing.

Benner, P. (1985). Quality of life: A phenomenological perspective on explanation, prediction, and understanding in nursing science. *Advances in Nursing Science, 1*, 1–14.

Black, G., & Haight, B. K. (1992). Integrality as a holistic framework for the life-review process. *Holistic Nursing Practice, 1*, 7–15.

Brallier, L. W. (1988). Biofeedback and holism in clinical practice. *Holistic Nursing Practice, 3*, 26–33.

Cousins, N. (1979). *Anatomy of an illness.* New York: W.W. Norton.

Dossey, L. (1982). *Space, time & medicine.* Boston: New Science Library.

Dossey, B. M. (1989a). The healer and the inward journey. In B. M. Dossey, L. Keegan, L. G. Kolkmeier, & C. E. Guzzetta, *Holistic health promotion: A guide for practice* (pp. 37–50). Rockville, MD: Aspen Publishers.

Dossey, B. M. (1989b). Imagery: Awakening the inner healer. In B. M. Dossey, L. Keegan, L. G. Kolkmeier, & C. E. Guzzetta, *Holistic health promotion: A guide for practice* (pp. 155–186). Rockville, MD: Aspen Publishers.

Dossey, B. M. (1989c). The psychophysiology of bodymind healing. In B. M. Dossey, L. Keegan, L. G. Kolkmeier, & C. E. Guzzetta, *Holistic health promotion: A guide for practice* (pp. 53–67). Rockville, MD: Aspen Publishers.

Dugan, D. O. (1989). Laughter and tears: Best medicine for stress. *Nursing Forum, 1*, 18–26.

Fitzpatrick, J. (1983). A life perspective rhythm model. In J. J. Fitzpatrick & A. L. Whall (Eds.), *Conceptual models of nursing: Analysis and application* (pp. 295–302). Bowie, MD: Robert J. Brady.

Gibson, Q. (1960). *The logic of social inquiry.* London: Routledge & Kegan Paul.

Guzzetta, C. E. (1989). Music therapy: Hearing the melody of the soul. In B. M. Dossey, L. Keegan, L. G. Kolkmeier, & C. E. Guzzetta, *Holistic health promotion: A guide for practice* (pp. 187–208). Rockville, MD: Aspen Publishers.

Hare, M. L. (1988). Shiatsu acupressure in nursing practice. *Holistic Nursing Practice, 3*, 68–74.

Kist, K. O. (1992, October). *The research role of the clinical nurse specialist as a marketing tool*. Paper presented at the 7th annual clinical specialist symposium of the Hunter-Bellevue School of Nursing, City University of New York, New York.

Kolcaba, K. Y. (1992). Holistic comfort: Operationalizing the construct as a nurse-sensitive outcome. *Advances in Nursing Science, 1,* 1–10.

Krieger, D. (1979). *The therapeutic touch: How to use your hands to help or to heal.* Englewood Cliffs, NJ: Prentice-Hall.

Krieger, D. (1981). *Foundations for holistic health nursing practices: The renaissance nurse.* Philadelphia: J.B. Lippincott.

Levine, M. E. (1971). Holistic nursing. *Nursing clinics of North America, 2,* 253–264.

Moccia, P. (1986). Theory development and nursing practice: A synopsis of a study of the theory-practice dialect. In P. Moccia (Ed.), *New approaches to theory development* (pp. 23–38). New York: National League for Nursing.

Newman, M. A. (1986). *Health as expanding consciousness.* St. Louis, MO: C.V. Mosby.

Newman, M. (1979). *Theory development in nursing.* Philadelphia: F.A. Davis.

Parse, R. R. (1981). *Man–living–health: A theory of nursing.* New York: Wiley.

Quinn, J. (1988). Building a body of knowledge: Research on therapeutic touch. *Journal of Holistic Nursing, 1,* 37–45.

Rogers, M. E. (1970). *An introduction to the theoretical basis of nursing.* Philadelphia: F.A. Davis.

Rogers, M. E. (1990). Nursing: Science of unitary, irreducible, human beings: Update 1990. In E.A.M. Barrett (Ed.), *Visions of Rogers' science-based nursing* (pp. 5–11). New York: National League for Nursing.

Ruxton, J. P. (1988). Humor intervention deserves our attention. *Holistic Nursing Practice, 3,* 54–62.

Selder, F. (1989). Life transition theory: The resolution of uncertainty. *Nursing & Health Care, 8,* 437–451.

Titlebaum, H. M. (1988). Relaxation. *Holistic Nursing Practice, 3,* 17–25.

Vines, S. W. (1988). The therapeutics of guided imagery. *Holistic Nursing Practice, 3,* 34–44.

White, J. A. (1988). Touching with intent: Therapeutic massage. *Holistic Nursing Practice, 3,* 63–67.

Zahourek, R. P. (1987). Clinical hypnosis in holistic nursing. *Holistic Nursing Practice, 1,* 15–24.

9 Spirituality and Ethics in Nursing Theory

SPIRITUALITY AND ETHICS: THE SAME OR DIFFERENT?

In Chapter 7 we talked about the difference between healing and curing, noting that the terminology of healing was often applied in newer paradigms. Furthermore, many theorists saw curing as only a small component of healing. Healing often was applied to the person; curing, to the disease. We now find a similar situation in relation to spirituality and ethics. Although both notions concern morality—what is right and wrong—they connote different images, different ways of handling oneself in the world.

The term *ethics* is more in keeping with older theories and an older world view. It focuses on rights and duties, on equity and justice, often with a rule orientation. *Spirituality* is a term more often found in theories arising in New Age paradigms.

Although ethics calls forth an image of a code of acceptable behavior, spirituality calls forth an image of life lived and experienced in light of certain beliefs and sensitivities. Because the terms have been used in nursing, there is a tendency for discussions of ethics to be connected to problems and vulnerabilities—dangerous situations in which the nurse might do the wrong thing.

Spirituality, on the other hand, has been related to the joyous experiences of soul growth and connection with a higher good, however envisioned. We might call spirituality the larger term and ethics, the more limited one. This is not to say that there is no crossover in the vocabulary in nursing theories.

Watson (1988) has captured the difference in connotation in the following citation:

Barbara J. Stevens Barnum: NURSING THEORY:
ANALYSIS, APPLICATION, EVALUATION, FOURTH EDITION.
© 1994, 1990, 1984, 1979 J.B. Lippincott.

> A nurse may perform actions toward a patient out of a sense of duty
> or moral obligation, and would be an ethical nurse. Yet it may be false
> to say he or she cared about the patient. The value of human care and
> caring involves a higher sense of spirit of self (p. 31).

We begin our comparison and contrast of the two ideologies by
looking at the renewed focus on the spiritual aspects of nursing.

SPIRITUAL ASPECTS OF NURSING

Despite nursing's strong historical roots in religion, it has been a
long time since nurses (outside of religious schools and institutions)
talked about the spiritual side of nursing. In eras past when nursing
was striving to prove itself a science, even its language changed,
deleting earlier references to spiritual values. As Donley (1991) said,

> Doctors acted like scientists, businessmen, or entrepreneurs. Nurses
> were also co-opted by the glamour and power of high-technology nurs-
> ing. As some of the art and most of the mystery of healing were lost, it
> became clear to nurses, and others who worked in hospitals, that they
> were part of a technical money-making system, not a "sacred system"
> (p. 178).

In the past two decades, older descriptions of nursing as caring
for the mind, body, and spirit were typically replaced by references
to biopsychosocial man. True, there were diseases of the body and
mind, but no one referred to diseases of the spirit. Few theories of
nursing involved the idea of spirit as an essential component. Only
a few schools of nursing (those affiliated with strict religious sects)
included courses on religion in their curricula or even required
church attendance. In these programs, religious values were frequently included in the life of the students, but seldom did religion
enter directly into nursing theory formulation. At best, one could
say that it formed an assumed context, an understanding that the
nurses in the organization would act out of spiritual motives.

Longway (1970), whose article was published in the *Journal of
Adventist Education*, was one of the few theorists who made a religious notion central to her theory. Working within a framework of
holism, she defined a circuit of wholeness in which man had unlim-
ited potential for growth and development, a wholeness denoting
harmony among parts (p. 21). To that notion she added the idea of
God as the source of man's power—power that could be cut off if a
man fell out of the plan of redemption (pp. 21–22). Disease was a
stoppage in man's power, and healing was the restoration of power
by providing energy:

The method whereby energy is made available to man is by giving, motivated by love, for giving completes the circuit of God, the source of power. . . .

The aim of intervention is to supply energy to the individual, help him to lay hold of more energy for himself and thus to enable him to advance along the illness-wellness continuum as far as his limitations will permit (p. 22).

Notice how close this description comes to some of the more modern works, especially theories related to New Age paradigms. Because Longway's nurse heals by supplying energy, the theory is one in which the nurse is a healer as well.

SPIRITUALITY IN NEWER NURSING THEORIES

Longway's theory was published more than 20 years ago, but it did not start a spiritual resurgence. That had to wait until the emergence of a new world paradigm. Now nurses are looking at spirituality again, and struggling to define the concept. Newman (1989) has noted that *holy, whole,* and *heal* all come from the same root meaning (p. 1). Hover-Kramer (1989) also has sought to locate spirituality in the search for wholeness and the surrender to a reality greater than ourselves (p. 29). Her position is much like that of transpersonal psychologists who see the spiritual as an emergent stage of growth.

Clark, Cross, Deane, and Lowry (1991) have noted nursing's inexperience with the spiritual dimension:

The process of defining spiritual care and spiritual needs has been elusive at best. It is not sufficiently developed to provide students and practitioners clear direction in strategies for using it in an intervention or for measuring spirituality as a part of quality care (p. 68).

Clark et al. (1991) have made clear their belief that a spiritual element in needed in nursing:

Spiritual well-being, the integrating aspect of human wholeness is characterized by meaning and hope. Quality care must include a spirit-to-spirit encounter between caregiver and patient. That includes the patient's acknowledgement of trust in the caregiver (p. 68).

From interviews, Clark et al. (1991) identified five major spiritual interventions as reported by patients:

1. establishing a trusting relationship
2. providing and facilitating a supportive environment
3. responding sensitively to the patient's beliefs
4. integrating spirituality into the quality assurance plan

5. taking ownership of the nurse's key role in the health care system (pp. 74–75).

The list may prove the authors' own point concerning the lack of work in this arena. Many of the items appear to be good nursing dictates, whether or not spirituality is involved. Indeed, spirituality may be a difficult concept to pin down because some associate it with religion, some with an attitude toward life, others with an advanced level of human development.

Traditional Religious Influences

Not all of the renewed focus on spirituality comes from theories using a new world paradigm. Traditional religious perspectives are also undergoing a renewed interest within the nursing community. These changes, however, are more recognized in changing nursing practices than in new theories. One such change is a new practice called *parish nursing*, a resurgence in nursing closely tied to a church or religious organization. Although the linkage between nursing and churches has been preserved over the years in many African-American churches, little about that practice has been written in nursing journals.

The new movement of parish nursing extends the practice to other churches and expands the position of the nurse beyond volunteer assistant during services. That is, a parish nurse is hired by a religious group to tend to its parishioners, or in some cases, to its geographic neighborhood. The parish nurse functions in much the same way that community health nurses function. About this resurgence, Smith (1991) has said,

> Parish nursing was born from the vision of Reverend Granger Westberg. Rev. Westberg worked as a hospital chaplain for many years, and his experience with nurses convinced him that they were "a national treasure." With one foot in the sciences and one foot in the humanities, Westberg believed nurses had great insight into the human condition (p. 28).

Smith related four generally accepted functions of the parish nurse in the new movement: (1) health educator, (2) personal health counselor, (3) trainee of volunteers, and (4) liaison with community resources (p. 28). So far, a unique *theory* of parish nursing has not been promulgated to my knowledge, although the functions of the role are being discussed in a practical exploratory manner.

Generally, it appears that the religious motivation is the *context* of nursing care rather than the content of the role. If parish nurses were used for religious proselytizing, one would have to ask the critical question: Is religious recruitment inherent in the theory of nursing? Or is the nursing role merely a vehicle to put a religious worker in touch with others for the purpose of proselytizing? In a Lutheran release, Martinson (1991) quoted Westberg as saying,

> A parish nurse is a much-needed "high-touch" component in the increasingly "high-tech" world of health care. In fact, insurers and government agencies should be singing the praises of parish nursing because it promotes preventive medicine, which is the least expensive form of health care (p. 2).

Here, it appears that the linkage is one of sympathy between the purposes of the church and nursing rather than an attempt to move the nursing ideology toward a spiritual base.

Substance Abuse Programs

One of the few arenas of care in which a spiritual component is more common than not in today's health is the treatment of alcohol and drug abuse. Typically these programs are multidisciplinary, not invoking the development of unique nursing theories. Most therapy models are based on the philosophy of Alcoholics Anonymous (AA), the first large-scale success in containing substance abuse. Bauer (1982) has claimed that the AA program succeeded by taking away moral guilt, offering hope, restoring dignity, and respecting individuality and the need to remain in the collective society (p. 25). The keystone of the AA program resulted from a letter by C. G. Jung to Bill W, one of the founders of AA. In that correspondence, Jung stated that he believed the abuse of alcohol to be a defective search for the spiritual. The cure for alcoholism, he said, was to be found in the spirit. Alcohol was the equivalent, on a low level, of spiritual thirst for wholeness; it represented the search for union with God (Bauer, 1982, p. 127). Jung added,

> You see, "alcohol" in Latin is spiritus, and you use the same word for the highest religious experience as well as for the most depraving poison. The helpful formula therefore is: spiritus contra spiritum (Cited in Bauer, 1982, p. 127).

The most successful approach in treating substance abuse so far, the 12-step AA program and its clones in drug abuse (e.g., Cocaine Anonymous and Narcotics Anonymous), have grounded recovery in a relationship to a higher power. In regaining this missing sense of spirit, the abuser regains his relationship to a higher power. There is no attempt on the part of these programs to link into a specific church or religion, yet the notion of a higher power is taken quite literally.

AA has taken the spiritual message to heart in an era that has pushed science as a substitute for God. Is substance abuse a natural backlash in a society seriously divorced from spiritual values? Is the rampant substance abuse of this age an ironic thwarted search for spirit as Jung believed?

Notice the verbal imagery involved. Is drug *intoxication* a poor man's spiritual *intoxication?* Is it coincidence that one *gets high* on drugs just as religions point *heavenward?* Or that many crack users claim they are hooked on another reality revealed by the drug?

Whether one agrees with Jung that the deficit is spiritual, mere body cure (namely withdrawal and detoxification) seldom works a cure in substance abusers. Effective rehabilitation programs discover that they must offer more than just a substance-free state. As Gold (1984) has said in relation to cocaine abuse, one must fill the cocaine hours—the time that was previous filled with thinking about the drug, purchasing it, using it, hanging around with fellow abusers (pp. 43–44). AA and its imitators fill the abuse hours with a spiritual focus.

Some purists object that this substitutes one addiction for an-other—if one grants such a thing as addiction to religion. Others protest that the AA programs themselves constitute an alternate ad-diction.

Clearly, the AA approach does not work for everyone. Nonbeliev-ers, for example, may object to the spiritual orientation. Others object to the sense of personal humility demanded in the surrender to a higher power. And loners may resent the close fellowship fostered among recovering substance abusers. Nevertheless, with all its limita-tions, the AA programs appear to run a higher rate of success than programs that do not address the spiritual element of the disease. That the AA ideology has been widely accepted by lay and multidisci-plinary professional leadership alike constitutes a strong recognition of the spiritual disease hypothesis.

Spiritualism in General Nursing Care

In addition to ever-increasing substance abuse programs, there has been a resurgence of attention to a spiritual dimension among tradi-tionally religious nurses. Within the Roman Catholic tradition, Sister Donley (1991) has suggested the following spiritual responses to patients' suffering: compassionate accompaniment, a search for meaning in the suffering, and action to remove the suffering. Here, then, is the beginning of a typology of spiritual care in relation to at least one concept: suffering.

As might be expected with any new aspect of care, there is a need to explore the domain before integrating it into practice. And the nature of spiritual care calls into question not only the nurse's knowledge of it but her personal qualifications to offer spiritual guidance. Nagai-Jacobson and Burkhardt (1989) and Stuart, Deckro, and Mandle (1989) have raised the problem of the nurse's own spiritual deficiencies and the inadequacy of her own spiritual resources. Indeed, their objection seems only fair. Few, if any, schools or employers take measure of a nurse's spirituality, nor do many set about to equip her for providing spiritual care.

New Age Spirituality and Nursing

We can anticipate more and more literature linking spiritualism and nursing as the New Age paradigm establishes itself. B. Dossey (1989) has identified three themes that locate the spiritual from this perspective:

1. the metaphysics that recognizes a divine Reality substantial to the world of things and lives and minds
2. the psychology that finds in the soul something similar to, or even identical with, divine reality
3. the ethics that place the human being's final end in the knowledge of the immanent and transcendent Ground of all being—the thing is immemorial and universal (p. 27).

Watson (1988) also considers spirituality an important component of nursing:

> The notion of a human soul is nothing new or original. It is, however, unusual to include it in a theory. The closest concept in psychology and nursing are concepts like self, inner self, "I," me, self-actualization, and so on. The bold attempt to acknowledge and try to incorporate a concept of the soul in a nursing theory is a reflection of an alternative position that nursing is now free to take. The new concept breaks from the traditional medical science model and is also a reflection of the scientific times. The evolution of the history and philosophy of science now allows some attention to metaphysical views that would have been unacceptable at an earlier point in time (p. 49).

Given nursing's early roots in religion, it is ironic that Watson has to search for permission to include aspects of the soul in a nursing ideology, yet it is impossible to dismiss her point. It is, indeed, the changing paradigm that encourages such inclusions. A major question not yet handled is just what nurses will *do* with the spiritual aspect of nursing where it is included, as well as how they will be judged qualified for the work involved.

Like Watson, Quinn (1992) invokes the sense of the spiritual when she speaks. Quinn has a unique conception of environment: the nurse as a healing environment for the patient, that is, the nurse as an energetic, vibrational field, integral with the client's environment. As she has said, the nurse should ask herself, " 'How can I become a safe space, a sacred healing vessel for this client in this moment?' " (p. 27) The nurse as a healing environment facilitates the multidimensional response of a whole person in the direction of healing and interaction. Obviously Quinn's view of reality is close to Watson's.

Similarly, Taylor and Ferszt (1990) have discussed spiritual healing in the new paradigm, defining *spiritual* as "that part of the self where the search for meaning takes place." (p. 32) They have addressed such esoteric methods as channeling, chakra therapy, past-life regression, rebirthing, breath work, color visualization, and crystal healing. Increasingly, one finds such New Age phenomena drifting into the nursing literature. Again the question is one of boundary: How is the New Age nurse different from other New Age advocates? Or, how is nursing spiritualism different from the function of other spiritual leaders?

Prince and Reiss (1990) also have struggled against the constraints of the scientific world view. In their case, they looked at how the model impacts on the labeling of persons as psychotic and on the care they subsequently receive. They noted that, from a different paradigm, some of these persons might be seen as normal. In many cultures, for example, the hallucinations of shamans are seen as sacred psychological states (p. 137).

Prince and Reiss (1990) have extended their perspective beyond shamanism to those labeled more frankly psychotic:

> In the Western world, when psychotics speak of their subjective experiences and the supernatural beliefs which often arise from them (delusions in psychiatric parlance), they are rejected by their more rationalistic confreres (p. 138).
>
> The usual reaction of the psychiatrist (but not necessarily of the lay reader) to ideas such as are expressed in this piece is to dismiss them as delusional and psychotic. The psychiatrist will pay little attention to their contents, apart from noting their formal aspects and as having relevance to diagnostic criteria. . . .
>
> In dismissing these ideas as meaningless, the psychiatrist relegates highly significant experiences of the patient to limbo. Concerns that are of most importance to the patient are irrelevant to the psychiatrist. . . .
> For the psychiatrist, the explanatory model (EM) of the patient with respect to his or her experience is completely unrealistic and even more damaging, non-negotiable (p. 141).

New paradigms developing in nursing are certain to return us to a consideration of spiritual matters and their place in nursing. Some new models of nursing, such as Watson's, already incorporate notions of spirituality; others are certain to follow.

Most of the nursing theories that look at spiritualism come from a holistic perception. Indeed, for those that adopt a transpersonal psychology as a base, spiritual development may be a natural phase of self-evolution beyond the more traditional stopping point at self-actualization.

ETHICS IN NURSING

When one turns from spirituality to ethics (at least as the notion appears in nursing), there is a radical shift in orientation. We move away from the notion of lifting the human spirit upward to an ideology, often with a sense of burden, always with a sense of duty.

The study of ethics has always had particular importance to nursing theory because the majority of nursing theories prescribe how nursing ought to be enacted rather than how it is enacted. (We are into rule setting here—obligations, dictates—not joyful uplifting of spirit.)

Most theorists decree what the *good* nurse ought to do. They identify the assumptions out of which the good nurse ought to act. Even those theorists who write descriptive theory, such as Benner (1984), express values. Her collection consists of *excellent* exemplars, that is, practice anecdotes already judged to be good.

Sometimes the link between a theory and its underlying ethical system is not as tight as the author might wish. The older theories have more difficulty integrating ethics than the New Age theories in which the spiritual is an intrinsic aspect.

It is not unusual for a reader to find a theorist proclaiming an ethical underpinning only to discover that the espoused ethical stance is superimposed rather than intrinsic to the theory. Some would argue this to be the case for Roy's (1980) stimulus–response theory. The espoused value system seems to be a slogan rather than a principle that drives the theory. Indeed, Roy can hardly be faulted for the failure. Because a stimulus–response theory represents the most mechanical (or scientific) view of man, it may be virtually impossible to overlay it with a religious passion.

Ethical Quandaries

Unlike the spiritual nursing focus, the ethical focus often fixates on problems. Often they involve exigencies of the practice setting, such as issues that arise out of tensions between cost control and quality of care or between quality of life and technology.

Ethical positions look at the nurse from a behavioral viewpoint, namely, considering what she ought to *do*. Here, we are addressing the notion of ethics as rule giving—controlling. From this perspective, the practice arena engenders an ever-increasing number of ethical questions and few definitive answers.

In the rule-giving orientation, ethical quandaries arise when changes in the environment confront people with new choices about what is right or wrong. The linkage with law rears its head, as decisions about new procedures and practices slowly are codified into laws and regulations. Today's health care environment is rampant with examples of such equivocal situations.

Sometimes the issue is economics. New technologies and new health care products have increased the range of health care options, yet the cost of these innovations often exceeds the ability of the society to pay for them. Society must decide which options will be developed and which will not, and it is a decision governing bodies seem reluctant to make.

One of the major problems from the ethical viewpoint is how to resolve the tension between a continuously developing science whose technology prolongs life versus the cost to society. Notice that this conflict occurs only when one accepts two normative sets of values: (1) the medical ideology that prolonged life of any quality is a prime value and (2) the socioeconomic preference not to place a major fiscal investment into the health care of people.

A nurse holding a New Age ideology might find this whole problem beside the point. She might argue that prolonging life is not itself a very important goal, that, indeed, it might obstruct the soul-development of persons who have elected to experience lives cut short at a young age. Indeed, she might consider the markers of life and death to be rather inconsequential in the longer view of a soul's development over various lifetimes.

The point to be made here is that ethics are very much tied to a nurse's world view. One's accepted world paradigm will ultimately dictate what nursing theories will appeal and what theories will not. In the past era, when most nurses in this culture shared the same world, even different ethical positions could be discussed from a common beginning point. That is no longer the case in nursing.

Quality of Life

Even under the older normative ideology, changes are coming about in ethical values. The increased respect for quality of life is a good example. Quality of life is the first value to confront head-on the medical assumption that preservation of life is always to be desired.

Nurses are more comfortable than physicians with decisions to allow certain patients to die. Currently, greater numbers of patients and their families are demanding their rights in the decision-making process. What was once settled by an authoritarian physician has become a negotiation in which many persons have a stake and in which life-at-any-cost is no longer seen as the right answer.

The ethical dilemma is complicated by the legal issue, that is, the vulnerability of those who take measures to stop or prevent life-preserving therapy. The court ideology is slow to change, following, not leading, normative practices in the society.

Equity in Health Care

The issue of equity is also problematic in the ethical decision-making paradigm. Most reasonable people would agree that health care should be equitable, yet what constitutes equity is not so simple. One party's equity is another's deprivation.

What about the inequity when parents from different social strata, with different means, compete for a scarce resource, say a liver for a dying child? What about the rights of a financially stressed surrogate mother versus the rights of the wealthy contracting father? What about the rights of their child? What about the terminal patient seeking to discontinue life support in the face of family opposition? What about a reduced population of young people carrying the tax burden for a disproportionate number of old and old-old people in the general population? What about those who are denied health care access because they lack the ability to pay? The problems of equity expand to tomes with little effort.

The cases and causes are numerous, but in each example, one asks, Who decides? Who pays? Who has rights? Who has obligations? What is justice? The problem in making most of these decisions is that the choices do not involve choosing between right and wrong, good and bad; instead, they involve choosing between opposing goods. When one discusses morality in terms of rights, justice, and equity, the argument hinges on the older world view.

When Nurses Confront Ethical Issues

Ethical issues arise for the nurse in the old perspective in several ways. Zablow's (1984) study reported that nurses were caught between physician demands and actions they believed to be right for the patient. In such situations, the nurses felt pressured to yield to the physician's decree because of his perceived power in the institution. Additionally, some nurses feared that their organizations would not support them for ethical stands taken on disputable issues. In some cases, unfortunately, the dominant norms of the organization were such that nurses were not expected to challenge medical or organizational decisions. In these circumstances, the nurses felt powerless to exercise control, even over their own behavior.

In regular nursing practice, issues having ethical implications surface with regularity. They include but are not limited to do-not-resuscitate practices, management for suspected child abuse, patients' rights to informed consent, patients' rights to privacy and confidentiality, and the patient's right to die. These examples are only some of the more blatant issues.

In addition, it is impossible for the nurse using a holistic New Age theory to avoid dealing with these issues, because she is in a world of action just as much as is the nurse holding an older ideology. Of course, none of these issues can be altogether resolved by a policy statement. Reasonable people may disagree on principles and even on actions when they agree on principles.

Sometimes the real moral dilemmas arising for nurses relate not so much to hard ethical choices, but to options forgone because of limitations on staff and resources. Financial stringency may be necessary for an institution's survival, but many nurses face quandaries of conscience when they see needy patients turned away because of inability to pay. Others face moral dilemmas when the situation simply allows them insufficient time to meet critical patient needs.

Institutional Solutions

Most institutions attempt to deal with ethical problems by a committee route. An ethics committee decides on the best action in serious, ambiguous cases with ethical and legal overtones. Such committees function to prevent arbitrary and premature decision making in complex cases. Even with a committee, however, there may be honest moral disagreements on the best way to handle a given problem. The use of deliberative, committee decision making offers some legal protection. Legal judgments may be sought in particularly complex circumstances.

An institutional review board serves as another clearinghouse for ethical problems—those that arise in medical, nursing, and other research endeavors that use patients as subjects. Even though such committees may be composed of people holding different beliefs, there is merit to joint deliberation. The quality of decision making certainly is improved by a thoughtful contemplative process.

The interplay of ethics and research has always been an important issue for nurses. Munhall (1988), for example, discussed the way in which the therapeutic imperative (i.e., patient advocacy) must take precedence over the research imperative. In Munhall's view, informed consent must be seen as dynamic and ongoing, hence invalidated if the circumstances under which the consent was gained change.

Ethical Guides

It is of value for any nurse to understand the norms of her society regarding ethics and ethical judgments. This is true whether or not the nurse personally comes from the same ideology. Probably the greatest change in recent years has been the growing involvement of people in their own health care. Acceptance of the patient's right to participate in full and informed decision making regarding his condition, prognosis, and treatment is a major aspect of this involvement.

The President's Commission for the Study of Ethical Problems in Medicine and Biomedical and Behavioral Research (1982, pp. 15–68) stressed patient autonomy as one of its hallmarks. This emphasis reflects a change in the normative society's way of perceiving the relationship between patient and health care professional.

The American Medical Association (1984) Judicial Council wrestled with the ethics of medical practice, addressing numerous issues of complexity ranging from ethical business practices for physicians to physician–patient relations. This body even formulated criteria for patient access to scarce resources in cases of necessary rationing. The document stated that:

> limited health care resources should be allocated efficiently and on the basis of fair, acceptable and humanitarian criteria. Priority should be given to persons who are most likely to be treated successfully or have long term benefit. Social worth is not an appropriate criterion (p. 3).

The nursing profession lacks such a judicial board, but it has a published code of ethics. The American Nurses Association's (1985) Code for Nurses provides guidelines concerning nurses' obligations to patients, colleagues, and the larger society. It does not, except in the broadest of terms, address specific ethical dilemmas such as access to health for the uninsured and homeless, abortions, do-not-resuscitate orders, medical experimentation, distribution of scarce health resources, or allocation of expensive technology. In addition, it cannot tell the nurse what to do in particular situations. The code is a useful guide, but ethical decisions still need to be puzzled out in light of the unique situational variables in each case. In essence, the code falls prey to the flaws in any system that attempts to dictate concrete, specific actions by generalized rules of behavior.

A PHILOSOPHICAL OVERVIEW OF ETHICS

In addition to the practical differences in the two notions of valuing most dominant in nursing (the traditional ethics focus and emerging notions of spirituality), one can consider the differences among ethical positions as perceived through a philosophical approach. The first differentiation is between a philosophy of *determinism* and one espousing human *freedom*. In determinism, all things happen in terms of antecedents. If one knew what had happened in the past, one could predict a present action. In this belief system, man has no free will; consequently, ethics do not exist. If all choices are the inevitable result of earlier events, then one cannot be morally accountable for his acts. To allow for ethics, there must first be some freedom of choice; one must be able to choose right over wrong.

Even among theories that espouse human freedom of choice and will, there are two positions; in one formulation, *ethical choice* exists; in the other, *moral skepticism* holds forth. The moral skepticism position claims that, although people are free to choose, the choices they make are not influenced by ethics. Moral choice is illusory in moral skepticism; ethics is an empty word. People choose all right, but not on the basis of what is good or bad.

Among those positions that support the existence of ethics in choosing, we can make yet another differentiation—one based on the way in which something is known to be ethical. Here, one asks, What makes an act ethical? Again there are two possible answers: *teleologic* or *deontologic*.

Teleology refers to the end, result, or goal. Teleologic systems place ethics in one of two final loci (making another set of options). Some teleologic positions judge an act ethical according to its *intentions*. Others judge an act ethical according to its *consequences*. The same act can be ethical in one system and unethical in another. Suppose a professor passed a borderline student to be kind (intention). Suppose, furthermore, that the student's ignorance in the subject matter caused the death of a patient (consequence). The act of the professor (passing the student) would be judged differently by persons holding these alternate teleologic positions.

The deontologic position judges an act, neither by its intentions nor its consequences. Instead, it judges an act to be ethical based on its conformity with something else. That something else, as one might suspect, varies from philosophy to philosophy. Three common options might be (1) the *laws* of the society; (2) *God* (or His revealed word, however conceptualized); or (3) one's *conscience.*

Let us look at just one of these options—conscience—to illustrate the complexity. In using one's conscience, the problem is that different consciences dictate different acts. Furthermore, there are many different interpretations of conscience. Some see it is a *learned response.* One might, for example, place Freud's internalization of the superego in this category. A second interpretation of conscience might be that it is the *law of reason.* Here, one might refer to logical rules such as Kant's (Behler, 1986) categorical imperative (pp. 53–125). Another interpretation finds conscience in *sentiment;* the inner voice theory might represent this view—whatever feels right.

For one last differentiation, let us look at the notion of sentiment. If one responds to an inner voice, it is still possible to ask how that inner voice makes its decisions. Does it intuit that certain *rules* are good, for example, never tell a lie, do not commit murder? Or does the sentiment function to judge each act separately? If it judges acts separately, then it might be right to murder in one case (when the ax murderer is attacking one's children), but not in another case.

This rather incomplete analysis of the nature of ethics and the meaning of ethics for persons holding different philosophies of life is intended only to make the nurse cognizant of the complexity of the subject. People of good will, all of whom identify themselves as moral, may disagree in good faith.

COMPARING PERSPECTIVES

The inherent conflict between a rule-oriented, rights-and-duties concept of ethics and a larger spiritual perspective might lend light to the ongoing dispute in nursing between the perspectives of Kohlberg (1981) and Gilligan (1982) on moral development. The application of Kohlberg's classificatory system for moral development was much used under the more traditional conception of ethics. The system typifies the view of ethics described here: rule bound, dealing with concepts of justice and equity. Numerous nurse researchers used his schema. But women in general and nurses in particular did not test well under Kohlberg's highly formal and abstract system.

The premises for Kohlberg's system was challenged by Gilligan (1982), who claimed that female morality is derived from personal relationships rather than abstract concepts. Although Gilligan certainly does not come from a New Age ideology, her work shows that the notion of ethics need not be limited to the older models. Huggins and Scalzi (1988) discussed this issue (among others) in their general review of ethical models.

Ethics and the new spiritualism often seem to arise out of different conceptions of the world. They present different problems, goals, values, and approaches. What they share is a focus on values and the need to negotiate between personal beliefs and societal norms.

SUMMARY

Nursing has an interesting history of intertwining with spirituality. One might say that nursing had its origin in religion. Much of our early history concerns nurses dedicated to the profession because of a religious commitment—usually to a codified belief system set in the context of a given religious sect.

Along the way, the religious origins of nursing were lost, some would say systematically sacrificed in the name of professionalism and scientific method. Even nursing schools sponsored by religious institutions frequently failed to include aspects of spirituality in the curriculum of care giving. In the practice setting, spirituality becomes the domain of the chaplain, not the nurse.

Then, in modern times, morality again reared its head, spurred by the ethical quandaries and legal problems created by the advancement of technology and the impositions of a suit-prone society. The study of ethics returned to nursing as an administrative or legal necessity. The focus was on helping patients make difficult care decisions or protecting the nurse and the institution from malfeasance.

Newer theories of nursing, those cast in a New Age ideology, present a different view of morality, one based in spiritual or developmental values. At present, both of these aspects (ethics and spirituality) are at play in nursing. While they are not necessarily at odds with each other, they certainly represent different perspectives on their underlying concerns.

REFERENCES

American Medical Association. (1984). *Current opinions of the Judicial Council of the American Medical Association.* Chicago: Author.

American Nurses' Association. (1985). *Code for nurses with interpretive statement.* Washington, DC: Author.

Bauer, J. (1982). *Alcoholism and women.* Toronto: Inner City Books.

Benner, P. (1984). *From novice to expert: Excellence and power in clinical nursing practice.* Menlo Park, CA: Addison-Wesley.

Clark, C., Cross, J. R., Deane, D. M., & Lowry, L. W. (1991). Spirituality: Integral to quality care. *Holistic Nursing Process, 3,* 67–76.

Donley, R. (1991). Spiritual dimensions of health care: Nursing's mission. *Nursing & Health Care, 4,* 178–183.

Dossey, B. M. (1989). The transpersonal self and states of consciousness. In B. M. Dossey, L. Keegan, L. G. Kolkmeier, & C. E. Guzzetta, *Holistic health promotion: A guide for practice* (pp. 23–50). Rockville, MD: Aspen Publishers.

Gilligan, C. (1982). *In a different voice: Psychological theory and women's development.* Cambridge, MA: Harvard University Press.

Gold, M. S. (1984). *800-cocaine.* New York: Bantam Books.

Hover-Kramer, D. (1989). Creating a context for self-healing: The transpersonal perspective. *Holistic Nursing Practice, 3,* 27–34.

Huggins, E. A., & Scalzi, C. C. (1988). Limitations and alternatives: Ethical practice theory in nursing. *Advances in Nursing Science, 4,* 43–47.

Kant, I. (1986). Foundations of the metaphysics of morals. In E. Behler (Ed.), *Immanuel Kant: Philosophical writings* (pp. 53–125). New York: Continuum.

Kohlberg, L. (1981). *The meaning and measurement of moral development.* Worcester, MA: Clark University Press.

Longway, I. (1970). Toward a philosophy of nursing. *Journal of Adventist Education, 3,* 20–27.

Martinson, V. (1991). *Founder of parish nurse movement urges return to "high-touch" health care for a "high-tech" world* (October news release, pp. 1–4). Park Ridge, IL: Lutheran General Health Care System.

Munhall, P. L. (1988). Ethical considerations in qualitative research. *Western Journal of Nursing Research, 2,* 150–162.

Nagai-Jacobson, M. G., & Burkhardt, M. A. (1989). Spirituality: Cornerstone of holistic nursing practice. *Holistic Nursing Practice, 3,* 18–26.

Newman, M. A. (1989). The spirit of nursing. *Holistic Nursing Practice, 3,* 1–6.

President's Commission for the Study of Ethical Problems in Medicine and Biomedical and Behavioral Research. (1982). *Making health care decisions. Vol. 1: Report.* Washington, DC: U.S. Government Printing Office.

Prince, R. H., & Reiss, M. (1990). Psychiatry and the irrational: Does our scientific world view interfere with the adaptation of psychotics? *Psychiatric Journal of the University of Ottawa, 3,* 137–143.

Quinn, J. F. (1992). Holding sacred space: The nurse as healing environment. *Holistic Nursing Practice, 4,* 26–36.

Roy, C. (1980). The Roy adaptation model. In J. P Riehl & C. Roy (Eds.), *Conceptual models for nursing practice* (2nd ed., pp. 179–188). New York: Appleton-Century-Crofts.

Smith, P. K. (1991). The parish nurse. *Communique, 2,* 28–29.

Stuart, E. M., Deckro, J. D., & Mandle, C. L. (1989). Spirituality in health and healing: A clinical program. *Holistic Nursing Practice, 3,* 35–46.

Taylor, P. B., & Ferszt, G. G. (1990). Spiritual healing. *Holistic Nursing Practice, 4,* 32-38.

Watson, J. (1988). *Nursing: Human science and human care: A theory of nursing.* New York: National League for Nursing.

Zablow, R. J. (1984). *Preparing students for the moral dimension of professional nursing practice: A protocol for nurse educators.* Unpublished doctoral dissertation, Teachers College, Columbia University, New York.

BIBLIOGRAPHY

Bandman, E. L., & Bandman, B. (Eds.). (1978). *Bioethics and human rights: A reader for health professionals.* Boston: Little, Brown.

Blecher, A. E., Dettmore, D. R., & Sisson, R. (1989). Spirituality and sense of well-being in persons with AIDS. *Holistic Nursing Practice, 4,* 16–25.

Burkhardt, M. A. (1989). Spirituality: An analysis of the concept. *Holistic Nursing Practice, 3,* 69–77.

Chally, P. S. (1990). Theory derivation in moral development. *Nursing & Health Care, 6,* 302–306.

Cunningham, N., & Hutchinson, S. (1990). Myths in health care ethics. *Image, 4,* 235–242.

Curtin, L. L., & Flaherty, M. J. (1982). *Nursing ethics: Theories and pragmatics.* Bowie, MD: Robert J. Brady.

Domire, S. L. (1989). Models for moral response in care of seriously ill children. *Image, 2,* 81–84.

Haase, J. E., Britt, T., Coward, D. D., Leidy, N. K., & Penn, P. E. (1992). Simultaneous concept analysis of spiritual perspective, hope, acceptance and self-transcendence. *Image, 2,* 141–147.

Hoyer, P. J., Booth, D., Spelman, M. R., & Richardson, C. E. (1991). Clinical cheating and moral development. *Nursing Outlook, 4,* 170–173.

Klein, S. (1989). Caregiver burden and moral development. *Image, 2,* 94–97.

National League for Nursing. (1980). *Ethical issues in nursing and nursing education.* New York: Author.

Nokes, K. M. (1989). Rethinking moral reasoning theory. *Image, 3,* 172–175.

Packard, J. S., & Ferrara, M. (1988). In search of the moral foundation in nursing. *Advances in Nursing Science, 4,* 60–71.

Parker, R. S. (1990). Measuring nurses' moral judgments. *Image, 4,* 213–218.

Reilly, D. E. (1989). Ethics and values in nursing: Are we opening Pandora's box? *Nursing & Health Care, 2,* 90–995.

Rew, L. (1989). Intuition: Nursing knowledge and the spiritual dimensions of persons. *Holistic Nursing Practice, 3,* 56–68.

Thomas, S. A. (1989). Spirituality: An essential dimension in the treatment of hypertension. *Holistic Nursing Practice, 3,* 47–55.

Wilson, D. M. (1992). Ethical concerns in a long-term tube feeding study. *Image, 3,* 195–199.

Yeo, M. (1991). *Concepts and cases in nursing ethics.* Petersborough, Ontario: Broadview Press.

10 Principle, Interpretation, and Method

USE OF ANALYTIC DEVICES IN UNDERSTANDING THEORY

Chapters 1 and 2 presented six analytical devices for theory analysis:

1. using commonplaces to define theory elements and their interrelationships
2. determining the level of theory development (descriptive or explanatory)
3. discriminating nursing from nonnursing acts, that is, determining boundaries
4. locating the theory on a patient–interaction–nurse continuum
5. recognizing relevant underlying assumptions
6. recognizing slogans and selective perception.

Three further analytical devices are presented in this chapter: (1) description of theory as to principle, (2) interpretation, and (3) method. This system may be used instead of analysis by content, process, context, and goals, if the reader finds it useful. If it seems too complex, the other method is satisfactory for making most significant differentiations.

PRINCIPLE

Every nursing theory is based on one or more dominant principles. A *principle* is the crux of a theory, an idea that is essential for stating or explaining it. Depending on the author's way of thinking, a principle may be presented as a starting point or as an ending point.

Barbara J. Stevens Barnum: NURSING THEORY:
ANALYSIS, APPLICATION, EVALUATION, FOURTH EDITION.
© 1994, 1990, 1984, 1979 J.B. Lippincott.

Compare Hall (1966), discussed in Appendix A, and Orlando (1990) to illustrate these different approaches. Hall arrived at her basic principle of self-mastery at the end of a chain of reasoning, and she placed it at the end of her article. Orlando, in contrast, asserted her principle by the second page:

> *It is, therefore, exceedingly important for the nurse to distinguish be-*
> *tween her understanding of general principles and the meanings which*
> *she must discover in the immediate nursing situation in order to help*
> *the patient. In making the distinction, the nurse first attempts to under-*
> *stand the meaning to the patient in a time and place context of what*
> *she observes and how she can exercise her professional function in*
> *relation to it (Orlando, 1990, p. 2).*

Orlando then used the rest of the book to better clarify and explain the principle through a more complete description and numerous examples of how it functions. Most authors follow one of these two patterns: (1) working toward a final discovery of the principle(s) or (2) stating the principle(s) and then explaining the ramifications.

Because nursing theories usually deal with both patients and nursing acts, it is not unusual to find *complementary principles,* one residing in the patient and one in the nursing act. For example, Hall's principle of self-mastery in the patient is complementary to the principle of mirroring in the nursing act. Similarly, Orlando's nurse tells what she sees, and the patient confirms or disconfirms its meaning.

Not all principles rest in the patient or the nursing act. Some principles rest in other aspects of the situation. For example, King's (1981) principles (action, transaction, and interaction) are found in the relationship itself rather than in either the patient or nurse.

One should identify each key principle of a theory, then consider the *nature* of each principle. Compare, for example, Hall's (1966) patient-based principle of *self-mastery* with Levine's (1971) patient-based principle of *adaptation.* For Hall, the principle rests in the agent himself. (Hall said that the patient *chooses* ill behavior or well behavior.) This sort of principle is termed *actional:* the principle is part of the agent. Notice that self-mastery (for Hall) can occur in a patient with little control over his own body or environment. Indeed, self-mastery may occur (or fail to occur) in favorable or unfavorable circumstances. Actional principles typically are found in human drives, motives, needs, or intentions.

Levine's adaptation principle, on the other hand, is located in the interaction of agent and circumstance. Adaptation means a constant adjustment of the individual to his changing environment (circumstances). This sort of principle is termed *reflexive.* Reflexive principles in nursing are often characterized by states of homeostasis, equilibrium, or exchange.

The difference between actional and reflexive principles can be illustrated by contrasting two additional theories. Flaskerud, Halloran, Janken, Lund, and Zetterlund (1979) presented a nursing theory that is unusual in that it is based on observation of *what is*, instead of *what ought to be*. In multiple observations of nurses working in diverse settings, the authors found two consistent principles at work: *avoidance* and *distancing*. These are actional principles because they describe behaviors located in the agent (in this case, the nurse). The behaviors were exhibited consistently without being altered in kind by the settings or patients involved. The actions were *by* the nurse, *for* the nurse.

In contrast to Flaskerud et al., Orlando (1990) has a reflexive principle. The nurse observes a specific patient behavior that she believes has significance. She identifies the behavior and verbally reflects it back to the patient with her interpretation of what the behavior means. The patient then corrects any misinterpretations before the nurse acts on them. The nurse cannot make a final judgment without the patient's input. When the behavior is called to the patient's attention, if he had not previously recognized the behavior, this mirroring back enables him to reflect on the behavior and its meaning. Interaction theories such as Orlando's often involve a reflexive principle.

There are two other types of principle: *comprehensive* and *simple*. The comprehensive principle explains a phenomenon by reference to a larger whole. For example, one might explain why a child is unable to perform a given psychomotor task by reference to the principle of *learning readiness*. Notice that learning readiness is a larger notion than the specific task failure that it explains. The same principle of learning readiness might explain hundreds of other task failures as well as task achievements. The principle of learning readiness is overarching, larger, and more comprehensive than those specific instantiations of it.

One might, on the other hand, have attempted to explain the child's failure in the psychomotor task by reference to the absence of the requisite series of stimulus–response patterns in his behavior. Here, the explanation directs attention to component parts of the phenomenon rather than to some overarching whole. Principles of this sort are termed *simple*. A simple principle explains a phenomenon by reference to its component parts (i.e., to its elemental building bricks). To explain man as so many interacting atoms uses a simple principle, whereas to explain man as an instantiation of a moving life process uses a comprehensive principle.

Rogers (1970) uses comprehensive principles. In her early work, she explained man by reference to the principle of reciprocy, a principle that relates man to his environmental field (p. 97), that is, a larger entity encompassing man and environment.

Like Rogers's theory, Newman's (1986) has a comprehensive principle. Newman has identified health, the goal of nursing, as the expansion of consciousness (p. 33). But expansion of consciousness does not simply mean learning new things or becoming more adept at one's cognitive or affective functions. Instead, expansion of consciousness involves actual change in what one is, in the patterning that is the essence of a man's being. The goal of nursing is to move man toward becoming, toward a higher level of existence and awareness. The principle of expansion of consciousness represents a greater whole than the present man.

Roy's (1980) theory, in contrast to the theories of Rogers and Newman, uses a simple principle, explaining man on the basis of stimulus, response, and adaptation levels. The stimulus and response are parts of the phenomenon being explained; they do not constitute a whole larger than man.

In summary, principles may be given as starting or ending points of a theory; they may reside in patient, nurse, or situation; and they may be actional, reflexive, comprehensive, or simple, a system of analysis borrowed from McKeon (undated, 1954). A principle is a fundamental or basic concept with an explanatory function, revealing the basis on which the theory is built. It is the fulcrum on which the rest of the theory depends.

INTERPRETATION

To determine interpretation in McKeon's system, one asks, What is reality (or the reality of the phenomenon under consideration) really like for the author? The reader will recognize this as identical to what we earlier called context. Examining the meanings given to the major terms of the theory provides the best clue. The first differentiation is easy. Theorists perceive the essence of their subject matter to fall either within human experience (phenomenal) or beyond human experience (transcendental).

Where the theory places the subject of nursing within human experience (phenomenal), it is possible to further interpret that theory as either *existential* or *essential*. In an existential theory, the subject matter of nursing rests in the human agent's acts, ideas, or impulses. A nursing theory based on empathy or personal power, for example, would be interpreted as existential. Both empathy and power can be experienced directly, and both can be perceived as primarily personal to and for the agent experiencing them.

Note the existential world in which nursing occurs for Paterson and Zderad (1988):

> When I, nurse, respond in the arena of my lived nursing world, I respond to a particular person in this "here and now" with all my background and all my anticipation of the future (p. 57).
>
> To me, a nurse is a being, becoming through intersubjectively calling and responding in her suffering, joyous, struggling, chaotic humanness, always trying beyond the possible while never completely free from ignoble personal wants (p. 56).

In contrast, an essential interpretation is one in which the nursing phenomenon is explained by reference to the circumstance in which it occurs. For example, Arakelian (1980) has an essential interpretation when she proposes nursing actions based on a patient's locus of control. The patient with an internal locus of control sees himself in control of his own fate (or the events in his life); the patient with an external locus of control sees things as happening to him—by luck, fate, or through acts of a powerful other.

Arakelian has recommended shifting the patient with an external locus of control toward a perception of internal control to make him assume responsibility for his health and therapy. This theory has an essential interpretation because what constitutes the underlying reality is the patient's relationship to the world (controlling the world or being controlled by it).

It may be difficult to decide whether a phenomenal theory is existential or essential. Because nursing inevitably occurs in an extant setting, the reader may have a tendency to view all theories as essential. In assigning an interpretive category, one must look for predominance of perspective rather than for an absolute. One asks, How does this theorist really see the world of nursing? What perspective dominates? What meaning underlies the theorist's selected terms? Because many nurse theorists use the same terms, it is important to examine the meaning of terms within a given theory. Subtle shifts of meaning for the same term occur from one theorist to another.

Hall (1966), for example, might appear, at first glance, to have an essentialist theory. There is interaction with circumstance on the part of the nurse; she interacts with the patient and his body. But the theory is existential, not essential. The *significant* world in which Hall's nurse works is the world of person (i.e., the world of mind, awareness, and mastery).

Levine's (1971) concept of nursing, on the other hand, is context imbedded: the patient's adaptations involve response to and interaction with the environment. The same is true of the nurse: her environment is the patient himself, and the nature of her conservation measures depends on an accurate reading of his responses. Levine's theory, then, is essential in its interpretation.

Because nursing is an applied discipline, it might be expected that all theories would use one of the phenomenal approaches to interpretation. That is not the case. Transcendental interpretations (beyond experience) consist of two types: *ontic* and *entitative*. The ontic interpretation sees the nursing reality as larger than life, and hence *above* direct experience; the entitative interpretation sees reality as *reductive* (i.e., consisting of units that are microscopic or microcosmic). To describe human behavior by reference to nerve cells and synapses is an *entitative* interpretation. To describe human behavior by reference to life phases, or an evolving consciousness, on the other hand, is an *ontic* interpretation. Note that neither the nerve cell nor the life phase can be experienced in itself.

Neuman (1980) exemplifies an entitative approach to nursing theory by describing man in five multicomponents: (1) basic structure and energy resources (e.g., genetic structure, response pattern, organ strength, ego strength); (2) individual intervening variables (e.g., basic structure idiosyncrasies, natural and learned resistance, time or encounter with stressor); (3) stressors (similarly broken into component types); (4) lines of resistance; and (5) various other perceived elements (p. 120). Neuman's theory is entitative because it describes man (and nursing) by reference to simple elements.

Jones (1978) also has a transcendental, entitative theory. She has described reality as follows:

> Syntoxic responses trigger messengers that act as tissue tranquilizers, creating a passive tolerance that permits a kind of peaceful coexistence with aggressors. Catatoxic messengers stimulate active efforts to destroy the aggressor. Among the best-known syntoxic messengers are the anti-inflammatory corticoids. . . (p. 1902).

Syntoxic and catatoxic response-triggering messengers are smaller than that which they explain and are indirectly accessible to human experience.

One may contrast this with the ontic interpretation of Newman (1986):

> The last stage is absolute consciousness, which has been equated with love. In this state all opposites are reconciled. This kind of love embraces all experience equally and unconditionally; pain as well as pleasure, failure as well as success, ugliness as well as beauty, disease as well as non-disease (p. 47).

Here, man is described, not by reference to a reality of diverse components, but by finding the *whole* of being, in this case, participation in full consciousness. Newman's interpretation is ontic because what is *most real* for her is this transcendental state of being, most real even though we have yet to experience it.

Watson (1988), like Newman, embodies an ontic interpretation of man and reality:

> My conception of life and personhood is tied to notions that one's soul possesses a body that is not confined by objective space and time. The lived world of the experiencing person is not distinguished by external and internal notions of time and space, but shapes its own time and space, which is unconstrained by linearity. Notions of personhood, then, transcend the here and now, and one has the capacity to coexist with past, present, future, all at once (p. 45).

A nursing theory is perceived to be valid to the extent that it represents what seems most truly real to the theorist or reader. If the reader, for example, does not perceive Watson's transcendental world as the most real characteristic of life and of nursing, then she is not likely to accept the theory. Similarly, Roy's theory will not be accepted if the nurse cannot buy stimulus–response patterns as most representative of the world.

In a nursing theory, the interpretation reveals the setting, so to speak—the screen (or world) on which (or within which) the theory is played out. Interpretations may be ontic, entitative, essential, or existential, and they reflect an author's underlying perception of the character of nursing. They point out the location of the *real world* of nursing for each theorist.

METHOD

Not only can a theorist be characterized by her principles and interpretation, but she can be classified by the way in which she reasons. In examining how various theorists move from their givens (principles) to their conclusions, different thought patterns emerge. These can be termed *dialectic, logistic, problematic,* and *operational.* McKeon (undated) described these patterns in the following way:

> Among the numerous semantic schemes that have been used in philosophy, one persistent and useful organization has been built about differences of method. For all their ambiguity the differences between dialogue or the dialectical method, debate or the operational method, proof or the logistic method, and inquiry or the problematic method were stated in ancient philosophy, have run through histories of restatement and modification, and are still operative in contemporary philosophy (p. 3).

In analyzing method in a given theory presentation, one looks for the dominant thought pattern. For most well-developed theory statements, it is possible to identify a dominant thought pattern even if patterns are somewhat mixed.

Dialectic Method

The *dialectic* method works by taking as its perspective a whole that organizes everything else. The whole, however described, governs the relationships and provides coherence to the parts. The overarching organization is emphasized in this mode of thought. All components are parts of a larger whole, a whole that is different from and greater than a mere summation of those parts. The parts, taken together, do not exhaust the whole; the whole organizes the parts.

Reasoning in the dialectic method moves by *assimilation*. Contradictory views are resolved by progression to a higher level from which the contradictions are seen as compatible components in a larger unity. This form of reasoning assimilates apparently contradictory assertions into a higher statement—higher in that it encompasses the truth embodied in each of the lower statements (Fig. 10–1).

In nursing theory, Rogers (1990) is a dialectic thinker. Nursing is explained by reference to broader principles, those that explain man. Man in turn is explained by principles that characterize the universe. The movement of her principles reveals a dialectic pattern through these ever-expanding explanatory concepts. Her principle of integrality, for example, is the assimilation of human and environ-

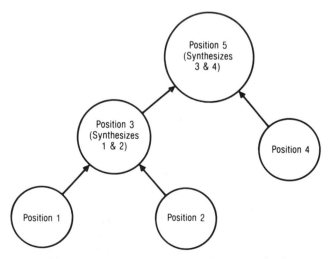

Figure 10–1. *Pattern in dialectic method.*

mental fields; her principle of helicy assimilates integrality with continuous innovative, unpredictable, increasing diversity (p. 8).

The welding of seemingly contrary fields is easy to identify in her (1970) older book:

> If the process of life is to be studied and understood, normal and pathological processes must be treated on a basis of complete equality. . . . The life process possesses its own unity. It is inseparable from the environment. The characteristics of the life process are those of the whole (p. 85).

Many nurses from an Anglo-American culture are unfamiliar with a dialectic mode of thought; hence, a philosophy such as that of Rogers tends to sound strange at first reading. She has both an unusual interpretation (e.g., energy fields and resonant wave patterns), and a less-used methodology (dialectic).

Smith (1981) applies a dialectic method to more common subject matter in examining the goal of nursing: health. She has identified four different conceptualizations of health: (1) the clinical model, (2) the role-performance model, (3) the adaptive model, and (4) the eudaimonistic model. After differentiating the models, she noted that each model may be subsumed under the next more comprehensive model.

Hence, achievement of clinical health (physiologic, biologic health), is subsumed in the role-performance model that incorporates other elements in its goal of achieving social functioning. In turn, the role-performance model is subsumed in the adaptive model, which incorporates social function into a larger notion of growth and development in interaction with one's environment. Similarly, the adaptive model is subsumed in the eudaimonistic model, whose goal incorporates growth and development into a larger goal of self-actualization (pp. 43–50).

Logistic Method

The logistic mode of thought moves in an opposite direction from the dialectic. In this case, the whole is not used to organize the parts, but the parts are used to organize the whole. Thus, a system, event, or entity is organized by reference to its parts and their interrelationships. Reasoning in the logistic mode moves by construction, as piece is added to piece and relationship added to relationship. Logistic thinkers often are called system builders, because their method creates a structure that resembles a geometric proof, with increasingly complex rules being produced in the system. Each complex rule (or entity) can be broken down into the less complex rules (or entities) from which it was derived. These rules in turn can be broken into simpler and simpler and, finally, self-evident rules. The mode of thought moves from the complex phenomenon to be explained to the simpler component parts that compose it (Fig. 10–2).

A clear example of logistic method is illustrated in nuclear physics, in which all physical objects are characterized by reduction to basic elements and their interrelationships. Unlike the dialectic mode, the logistic method does not focus on how a given part fits in relation to the whole; logistic method is not concerned with assertions about how this particular atom fits into the total universe. Attention, instead, is placed on assertions concerning how parts interrelate with each other, how this atom of hydrogen relates to that atom of oxygen.

The logistic mode is evidenced in a search for relationships—spatial, temporal, and causal. Even if the content of a logistic system becomes extensive (e.g., nuclear physics explaining the whole physical universe), the construct still rests on an analysis of the parts and their relationships, not on an analysis from the viewpoint of the whole.

The logistic method of thought is popular in the Anglo-American culture, and many writers of nursing theory advocate a logistic system. Hardy (1973), for example, illustrated the logistic approach to theory development:

> *Laws are well-grounded and empirically confirmed hypotheses. They state a constant relation among two or more variables, each representing (at least partly and indirectly) a property of concrete systems. An example of a law is* E = Mc^2. *In the psychosocial area few, if any, laws exist. Laws are propositions asserting universal connection between properties. Hypotheses are much less well established (i.e., have less empirical support) than laws.*

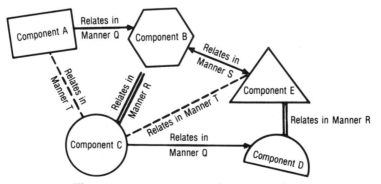

Figure 10–2. *Pattern in logistic method.*

> Statements on the highest level of generality are laws and axioms. Statements on a lower level of generality (theorems, hypotheses) can be deduced from laws. The reason for deducing these statements is to permit the general statements to be tested. In such a deductive system, high level statements can be falsified by the falsification of lower level (deduced) statements (p. 15).

The adoption of mathematic terms (e.g., axioms, propositions, laws) is not accidental. Indeed, mathematics is an ideal logistic method; its rules for interrelationships of particular variables (quantities) are highly specified, invariate, and closely bound in a unified system. Logistic theorists often aspire to reduce their theories to mathematics-like formulas.

Roy (1980) is a nurse theorist with a logistic method:

> The Roy Adaptation Model can be viewed primarily as a systems model though it also contains interactionist levels of analysis. The person as patient is viewed as having parts or elements linked together in such a way that force on the linkages can be increased or decreased. Increased force, or tension, comes from strains within the system or from the environment that impinges on the system. The system of the person and his interaction with the environment are thus the units of analysis of nursing assessment, while manipulation of parts of the system or the environment is the mode of nursing intervention. The person has four subsystems: physiologic needs, self-concept, role function, and interdependence (p. 179).

In this citation, Roy has addressed both components of her system, which are the component parts of man and the relationships among components (e.g., forces, tensions, and strains).

Johnson (1980) is another logistic nurse theorist; her subject matter (behavioral subsystems) differs from Roy's, but her methodology is similar:

> The subsystems are linked and open, as is true in all systems, and a disturbance in one subsystem is likely to have an effect on others. . . . Although each subsystem has a specialized task or function, the system as a whole depends upon an integrated performance (p. 210).

Johnson defines behavioral subsystems of attachment or affiliation, aggression, dependency, achievement, ingestion, elimination, and sex.

Problematic Method

The *problematic* method uses neither the parts nor some overarching whole as its basis. Instead, it acts by recognizing and defining unique problems, then reconciling the factors that constitute a given problem situation. In this sense, there is a *whole*, but the whole is different for any given problem; the whole contains the entirety of elements related to the problem and its solution. The problematic mode of thought differs from both the dialectic and logistic methods in that the problem solver himself is part of the method, that is, he is part of the circumstance in which the problem occurs. But for his identifying the situation as problematic, there would be nothing to initiate inquiry.

This involvement of the agent in the method is quite different from the way in which dialectic and logistic methods of thought function. The structure in these other methods is independent of the agent. The component parts of Roy's hypothesized man, for example, are unaltered by the agent applying her logistic method; in addition, the nature or ultimate nature of consciousness does not change from one of Rogers's nurses to another.

Reasoning in the problematic method aims at *resolution* through the interaction of the problem solver and the environment. The method is the familiar one of problem solving. Sometimes called the scientific method, problem solving involves the following five steps. The agent:

1. interacts with the environment by means of problem encounter.
2. enquires regarding the circumstances.
3. frames the hypotheses.
4. tests the implied consequences of the selected hypotheses.
5. confirms or rejects the hypothesis.

In the problematic method, problems may be linked: the solution to one problem becoming the means whereby another problem is investigated. The problematic method can present an evolving chain of related problems in which ends continuously are converted to means. Such a chain, however, does not terminate in a self-sufficient and bounded system as occurs in logistic and dialectic modes of thought. In the problematic method of thinking, each problem has its own universe, its own environment (those things that pertain to and have an impact on the problem). Problems arise only through the perception of an agent—the person who determines that a given situation is problematic. A problematic mode of thought is not directed toward fixed goal-achievement but rather toward resolution of the situation (Fig. 10–3).

The problematic approach is evident in the research of Burke, Kauffmann, Costello, and Dillon (1991). They first recognized a problem, noticing that

> disabled children not only had more hospitalizations, but also that hospitalizations were more stressful for "experienced" mothers of dis-

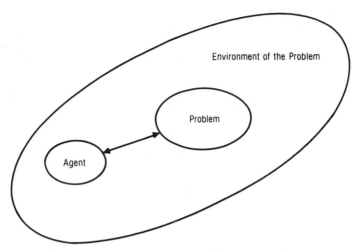

Figure 10–3. *Pattern in problematic method.*

abled children than for the less experienced mothers with nondisabled children. . . . The purpose of this study is to gain a better understanding of the stressful process for parents involved in repeated hospitalization of children with chronic conditions (p. 39).

Next, they search the *environment* of the problem—first, unsatisfactorily, the research. They found tangential reports, but nothing that dealt directly with their problem, so they expanded the notion of environment to include interviewing mothers of school-aged children with physical disabilities. They asked these mothers about their parental stress using a grounded theory approach. Grounded theory, incidentally, is a common method for problematic research because all the variables cannot be known at the start.

From these data, Burke et al. (1991) identified three types of incidents that increased stress: (1) negative information (information that turns out to be wrong); (2) gaps and variations in information; and (3) inexperienced health care workers practicing on their children. Burke et al. summarized these incidents as *hazardous secrets.* The parental response, termed *reluctantly taking charge,* was also found to contain three elements: (1) vigilance and covert taking over, (2) negotiation of rules and calling a halt, and (3) tenacious information seeking (p. 42). This is as far as the article went, but the problem-solving hypotheses can already be formed: If hazardous secrets increase, then parental stress increases.

Levine's (1971) early work was also problematic in approach. When one examines her conservation theory, her four conservation principles are really four separate problems to be solved by the nurse for every patient: How does one conserve energy? Structural integrity? Personal integrity? Social integrity? In typical problematic fashion, Levine treated each problem as its own separate universe with its own separate resolution. Unlike Roy or Johnson, for example, Levine did not attempt to interrelate the four principles (except insofar as they all addressed some aspect of conservation). She did not take a logistic approach, such as asking how conservation of social integrity might affect structural integrity or how conservation of energy might impact on personal integrity.

Moreover, she did not weld these concepts into some dialectic synthesis of an overarching whole. *Conservation* exists only through the concrete solving of the four separate problems. Each principle is addressed singularly, unmixed with issues of the other three conservation problems. In typical problematic thinking, Levine sees each problem in its entirety, with its own resolution. Also, as in typical problematic thinking, her system is unbounded; that is, further principles (i.e., problems) may be found in the future. It is interesting to compare Roy's (1980) concept of man with Levine's (1971). Their theory elements show some correspondence, as seen in Figure 10–4.

Despite their superficial correspondence, there is an important difference in the two sets of elements. Roy's elements are subsystems of man, but Levine's elements are located in the nursing act. Levine's four principles compartmentalize the nursing problems, not man. Therefore, Levine can assert a holistic view of man. Indeed, the whole man is the subject matter for each of her discrete nursing problems.

Compare the kinds of argument offered by Levine and Roy in support of their respective positions. Levine (1971) forwards her argument by giving numerous examples of each conservation principle in action. Because problem resolution differs slightly in every extant situation, this sort of argument is typical of a problematic thinker. Roy (1980), on the other hand, forwards her argument by reducing each component system of man into its subcomponents: stimuli (of three sorts); adaptation level; and response. Relations

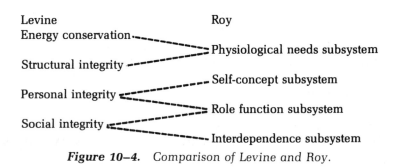

Figure 10–4.   *Comparison of Levine and Roy.*

among these more basic components are also discussed, completing the logistic linkages.

Operational Method

The *operational* method is similar to the problematic method in that the agent is part of the method. The problematic method involves an interaction between the agent and his environment; in the operational method, the perspective of the agent, rather than an interaction, determines the method. In a sense, the agent is the method, and this differentiates operational from problematic thought. Method cannot be independent of the perspective and activity of the agent in operational thought. Of course, a single person may have different perspectives at different times; and there are as many methods as there are different persons to perceive and use them.

Reasoning in the operational mode is typified in debate—one perspective versus another. Selection of one viewpoint over another may occur, but it is assumed that a plurality of views will remain. The operational method moves by *discrimination* between or among viewpoints; it unveils differences, usually by persuasion rather than formal proof.

Selection among viewpoints or between courses of action is not essential in all instances of the operational method; in some circumstances, there is no need for resolution. An operational nursing theory, for example, could present alternatives among which the reader might select according to his own preferences.

When systematic chains of reasoning occur in operational thought, movement occurs through choice among alternatives; either one perspective or another, one action or another, is chosen. *Either/or*, not synthesis, governs thought in the operational mode. Discrimination is the method used, and chains of reasoning are such that the alternative selected at the first point of choice constrains the alternatives available for choice at the second point in the chain. Whereas chains of reasoning in dialectic thought show synthesis (moving upward), a downward branching is discernible in operational thought (Fig. 10–5). At each step of operational thought, alternatives or finer and finer discriminations are identified.

In the operational method, the actions of the agent determine knowledge. For example, a foot (in length) in operational thought is not some absolute in itself; it is instead the operations of the agent that mark off a foot. An operational definition would not assert that a foot in one set of temporal–spatial coordinates is identical in length with a foot in another set of coordinates, but simply that the agent performs the same acts in each setting (i.e., the foot is defined by

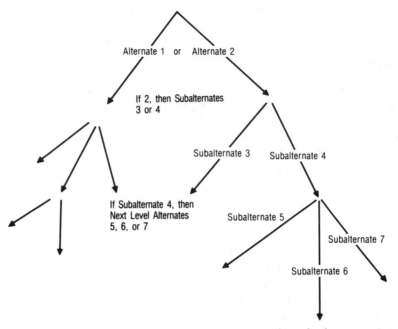

Figure 10–5. *Pattern in operational method.*

what is *done* rather than by what *is*). The methodology leading to knowledge rests in the action and the perspective of the agent. Orem (1985) is an operational thinker. Her argument moves by telling what the agent does—what discriminations the nurse makes among patient needs, what selection she makes among all modes of care. Orem's concept of self-care is the first entity subjected to operational differentiation. Self-care (an activity) is divided on the basis of who does it: *either* the patient *or* the nurse (pp. 38–39).

In typical operational fashion, Orem (1985) differentiates self-care into three types: (1) universal self-care requisites, (2) development self-care requisites, and (3) health-deviation self-care requisites (p. 90).

Orem further divides her major self-care categories according to specific areas in which the patient may need assistance. For universal self-care, Orem identified eight possible loci in which the patient may require help in the forms of maintenance, provision, or prevention:

1. intake of air
2. intake of water
3. intake of food
4. elimination processes and excrements

5. balance between activity and rest
6. balance between solitude and social interaction
7. hazards to life and well-being
8. human functioning and developing within groups (normalcy) (pp. 90–91).

Each segment of Orem's theory shows a similar operational pattern, in other words, breaks each concept into subordinate either/or options, making multiple layers of discriminations of one sort or another. Indeed, should one desire to do so, it would be possible to diagram Orem's book in an extensive series of downward branching chains of organization.

It is interesting that medicine has adopted an operational method for most of its education and practice whereas nursing has few operational theories. In medicine, the notion of *differential diagnosis* indicates the operational thought pattern. Although nursing process could be designed in an operational fashion, it is seldom so presented. Nursing process is usually presented in a logistic fashion.

Orlando's (1990) thought follows operational discriminations also. For example, she differentiates observations (raw material) into direct and indirect (p. 7) from which she draws consequences: to act or not to act (p. 8). Even her basic principle hinges on a difference: what is seen by the nurse, what is interpreted versus what is meant by the patient. If one examines her writing, the discriminating and selecting can be seen to resemble the same process applied by Orem.

THE READER'S TASK

The reader should bear in mind that (1) a principle is a statement that is key to how a theory works; (2) an interpretation is a statement as to *what* characterizes the circumstances (i.e., what reality is like); and (3) method is the characteristic manner in which an author thinks and organizes her assertions, statements, or arguments.

The reader is encouraged to read concurrently the theory works addressed in this chapter. This way, the analyses presented can take on meaning. Only in careful reading, rereading, and reasoned diagnosis will the reader develop the skills necessary for analyzing theories.

Not all theorists are consistent in the principles, interpretation, and method they apply. For example, a theorist may use a problematic method in one place, a logistic method in another. The best theories, however, are consistent. Confusion results in the reader's mind if the theorist arbitrarily switches back and forth, for example, between a physiologically based explanation of man (interpretation) and an explanation of man as psychological. If the reader has trouble analyzing a given theory, she should consider that the problem may be the author's inconsistencies.

ALTERNATE MODELS

Not all critics of theory use the strategy of analyzing principle, interpretation, and method; some have their own analytic tools. For that reason, the reader is advised to try several books that offer critiques of theory. Chinn and Kramer (1991), for example, suggest four structural devices for analytic purposes: (1) a triangle, (2) a circle, (3) a continuum, and (4) differentiation.

> The triangular drawing suggests that health is comprised of a series of related subconcepts that vary in breadth or simplicity. It also suggests foundational concepts upon which other subconcepts are built. . . .
> The overlapping circles depict discrete components that have common areas between and among them. . . .
> Applying this idea to the horizontal line drawing on the figure shows "health" represented as a continuum. This structure suggests that health is in a linear relationship with illness. . . .
> The fourth structural form conveys the ideal of differentiation, dividing major concepts into subconcepts (pp. 116–117).

Notice the relationship these structures bear to the materials discussed earlier in this chapter. The triangle, with broad foundational concepts on which more narrow notions are built, is virtually the opposite of the dialectic—in which reasoning starts with the narrow and moves to the broad. The second device (illustrated by a Venn diagram of three interlocking circles) does not represent any methodology discussed here, but certainly could be interpreted as a boundary demarcation. The third device, using a continuum rather than separation of opposing aspects, is often found in transcendental, ontic interpretations. Chinn and Kramer's final structure is essentially the opposite of their triangle image and roughly equivalent to the operational method as presented in this chapter.

Chinn and Kramer are not the only good critics of theory. The reader should also peruse books by Meleis (1991), Fitzpatrick and Whall (1983), and Walker and Avant (1988).

SUMMARY

The nurse who truly wants to understand theory needs to apply diverse analytic devices to her reading. This chapter has presented one such construct: the notion of a theory as a combination of principle, interpretation, and method. This method of analysis may be difficult for the nurse with little background in philosophy. Since it isn't the only method available to her, she shouldn't be concerned if she prefers other methods.

Nevertheless, taking a theory apart as to principle, interpretation, and method, even if the analysis is imperfect, will provide the reader with insight into what a theorist is doing. This exercise may be particularly valuable if the given theory appears abstruse or radically different from others she has studied.

REFERENCES

Arakelian, M. (1980). An assessment of nursing application of the concept of locus of control. *Advances in Nursing Science, 1,* 25–42.

Burke, S. O., Kauffmann, E., Costello, E. A., & Dillon, M. C. (1991). Hazardous secrets and reluctantly taking charge: Parenting a child with repeated hospitalizations. *Image, 1,* 39–45.

Chinn, P. L., & Kramer, M. K. (1991). *Theory and nursing: A systematic approach* (3rd ed.). St. Louis, MO: Mosby Year Book.

Fitzpatrick, J. J., & Whall, A. L. (1983). *Conceptual models of nursing: Analysis and application.* Bowie, MD: Robert J. Brady.

Flaskerud, J. H., Halloran, E. J., Janken, J., Lund, M., & Zetterlund, J. (1979). Avoidance and distancing: A descriptive view of nursing. *Nursing Forum, 2,* 158–174.

Hall, L. E. (1966). Another view of nursing care and quality. In K. M. Straub & K. S. Parker (Eds.), *Continuity of patient care: The role of nursing* (pp. 47–66). Washington, DC: Catholic University of America Press.

Hardy, M. E. (1973). The nature of theories. In M. E. Hardy (Ed.), *Theoretical foundations for nursing* (pp. 10–22). New York: MSS Information Corporation.

Johnson, D. E. (1980). The behavioral system model for nursing. In J. P. Riehl & C. Roy (Eds.), *Conceptual models for nursing practice* (2nd ed., pp. 207–216). New York: Appleton-Century-Crofts.

Jones, P. A. (1978). An adaptation model for nursing practice. *American Journal of Nursing, 11,* 1900–1906.

King, I. M. (1981). *A theory for nursing: Systems, concepts, process.* New York: Wiley.

Levine, M. E. (1971). Holistic nursing. *Nursing Clinics of North America, 2,* 253–264.

McKeon, R. (undated). *Philosophic semantics and philosophic inquiry* (mimeograph). Chicago: University of Chicago.

McKeon, R. (1954). *Thought, action and passion.* Chicago: University of Chicago Press. Concepts of principle, interpretation, and method as used in this book are taken from these organizing structures appearing in the various works of Richard McKeon.

Meleis, A. I. (1991). *Theoretical nursing: Development and progress* (2nd ed.). Philadelphia: J. B. Lippincott.

Neuman, B. (1980). The Betty Neuman health-care systems model: A total person approach to patient problems. In J. P. Riehl & C. Roy (Eds.), *Conceptual models for nursing practice* (2nd ed., pp. 119–134). New York: Appleton-Century-Crofts.

Newman, M. A. (1986). *Health as expanding consciousness.* St. Louis, MO: C. V. Mosby.

Orem, D. E. (1985). *Nursing: Concepts of practice* (3rd. ed.). New York: McGraw-Hill.

Orlando, I. J. (1990). *The dynamic nurse–patient relationship.* New York: National League for Nursing.

Paterson, J. G., & Zderad, L. T. (1988). *Humanistic nursing.* New York: National League for Nursing.

Rogers, M. E. (1970). *An introduction to the theoretical basis of nursing.* Philadelphia: F. A. Davis.

Rogers, M. E. (1990). Nursing: Science of unitary, irreducible, human beings: Update 1990. In E. A. M. Barrett (Ed.), *Visions of Rogers' science-based nursing* (pp. 5–11). New York: National League for Nursing.

Roy, C. (1980). The Roy adaptation model. In J. P. Riehl & C. Roy (Eds.), *Conceptual models for nursing practice* (2nd ed., pp. 179–188). New York: Appleton-Century-Crofts.

Smith, J. A. (1981). The idea of health: A philosophical inquiry. *Advances in Nursing Science, 3,* 43–50.

Walker, L. O., & Avant, K. C. (1988). *Strategies for theory construction in nursing* (2nd ed.). Norwalk, CT: Appleton & Lange.

Watson, J. (1988). *Nursing: Human science and human care: A theory of nursing.* New York: National League for Nursing.

11 *The Nursing Process and Problem Solving*

Nursing process and problem-solving theories are considered in the same chapter, not because they are alike, but because people so often confuse them. In fact, their structures are quite different. It is hoped the reader will appreciate this by the end of the chapter.

This is not to deny that the two theories are intermixed in some organizations, creating an inconsistent ideology. For example, a nursing service may require problem-oriented charting but simultaneously advocate the use of the nursing process. The basic incompatibility of these theories is discussed after each theory has been reviewed separately.

THE NURSING PROCESS

Often an incomplete theory evolves in the practice setting or nontheory nursing literature before it is recognized as a theory. This has been the case with the nursing process. It was highly popular in the United States before its theory implications were fully recognized. Its evolution toward full theory status has been occurring for more than two decades: first, development of the process itself, then, the addition of content elements (nursing diagnoses and nursing interventions) related to two steps of the process.

The term *nursing process* has been given many different meanings. Sometimes authors change the meaning of the term without even realizing it. The nursing literature commonly talks of *the* nursing process, not *a* nursing process, as if there were only one formulation. This is far from the truth, but for our purposes, we will work within a flexible description. However cast, the nursing process is a proce-

Barbara J. Stevens Barnum: NURSING THEORY:
ANALYSIS, APPLICATION, EVALUATION, FOURTH EDITION.
© 1994, 1990, 1984, 1979 J.B. Lippincott.

dure for organizing nursing care in which the first step (patient assessment) initiates the act of nursing. This step leads to the second step, which cannot be initiated until information has been garnered and processed in the preceding step. This format (each step depends on conclusions reached or acts completed in the prior step) continues through all the steps of the process until the last step (evaluation) is concluded. Often the information acquired at the final step completes a circle, starting the process again.

The content and number of steps in the nursing process account for the variability in definitions. Some formulations hold as few as four steps (assess, plan, implement care, evaluate); other formulations might have any number of the following steps:

1. patient assessment
2. nursing diagnosis
3. patient prognosis
4. goal setting
5. therapeutic care planning
6. care implementation
7. evaluation of
    a. patient status (reassessment post care)
    b. accuracy of prior assessment
    c. goal achievement
    d. accuracy of prognosis
    e. appropriateness of therapeutic choices
    f. effectiveness of care delivery
    g. needed alterations in the plan.

It is not uncommon for patient prognosis to be omitted in models of the nursing process. Similarly, evaluation often fails to consider the quality of the care implementation. In some formulations, the reassessment may be conceptualized as initiating a new nursing process rather than completing an ongoing one. For this discussion, the nursing process refers to the previously described process, whether or not its formulation includes all the possible logical steps.

Notice that the process is highly logistic. The format is a series of discrete components related to each other in unvaried sequence, prescribed and inflexible. For example, one never implements care before making a therapeutic plan; one never diagnoses before assessing. The very nature of the process forces its user to think in terms of interrelated components. Completeness means doing all the parts.

If one were to identify the process theory thread most dominant in nursing today, the nursing process would probably be that thread. Its use is prevalent in the standards of care published by the American

Nurses' Association (ANA), and it has also been adopted in large numbers of nursing schools and practice settings.

When one method of practice receives such extensive adoption, one must consider that the model has much to recommend it. That is certainly the case with the nursing process. First, it resembles the medical model and can be used for professional parallelism. Simply put, it is a way to assert that the nursing profession is just as mature as medicine. Of course, Henderson (1987), in an insightful article on the process, noted that parallelism may also mean separatism and failures in collaboration.

Perhaps the greatest appeal of the nursing process is that it offers a system for uniform practice. As with other logistic systems, the nursing process is unvaried, that is, designed so that any nurse applying it correctly comes to the same conclusions as any other—at least that is the ideal to be desired. In a profession seeking some measure of certainty, this aspect of the system appeals.

Because it encourages uniformity of practice, the nursing process enhances the possibilities of research, especially research applying quantitative measures. A strong commitment to this method of research on the part of many nurses may account for the system's popularity.

Extensive adoption of the nursing process also may indicate the process's superiority over other formats. Only time will tell. At the moment, one might say the glow of newness is wearing off, and there are major disagreements about its efficacy.

Additionally, holistic theories are vying for serious attention. Holistic theories and the nursing process represent the two strongest competitors in the theory business, and they represent virtually opposite ends of the pole as to principle, method, and interpretation. Kobert and Folan (1990) have given an excellent recounting of the points of disagreement in these two methods and their underlying philosophies.

Another reason for the popularity of nursing process is its adaptability. As a theory thread, the logistic nursing process is compatible with the many other logistic systems on the present health care scene (such as computer-generated management and information systems). For a generation of nurses raised on computers, the nursing process feels comfortable.

It is no coincidence that many of our leaders most heavily committed to the nursing process (and evolution of a related set of diagnostic labels) are the same people actively involved in the effort to identify a minimum nursing data set (the objective of which is to allow institutions to collect uniform data; see Werley & Lang, 1988).

Both systems are logistic with similar world views; both focus on nursing as a science in which nurses can replicate both judgments and research findings of their colleagues. In other words, these are systems designed to be universal in their application.

Although it is logistic, the nursing process is a *process* rather than a *content* element. It has the appeal of telling the nurse what to do. The process element is the weak link in many extant nursing theories, so it is not surprising that nurses are pleased to find a promising process.

LIMITATIONS

This is not to say that the nursing process has no flaws; every system has its limitations. Benner (1984) recognized an important one. Using the Dreyfus Model of Skill Acquisition (Dreyfus & Dreyfus, undated), she constructed a model of nursing research designed to explore clinical excellence. The Dreyfus model describes five separate levels of skill acquisition; and Benner, accordingly, differentiated nursing practice into these five levels. The five levels are

1. novice
2. advanced beginner
3. competent performer
4. proficient performer
5. expert.

Briefly, the levels can be characterized in the following way. The novice learns context-free rules to guide her actions. She gains few subtleties in understanding; she simply applies the objectifiable rules. The advanced beginner starts to appreciate some "aspects of the situation" that require prior experience for recognition. The advanced beginner still needs help in setting priorities and sorting out what is important from what is not. She is only beginning to recognize recurrent meaningful patterns.

The competent performer (a level reached after 2 to 3 years of practice) begins to see her actions in terms of long-range goals and plans. She lacks speed and flexibility but has a feeling of mastery and the ability to cope with many contingencies. The proficient performer sees situations as wholes rather than as concerned with isolated aspects. She recognizes when the expected picture fails to materialize and no longer relies on rules or analytic principles. Instead, she has an intuitive grasp of each situation and zeroes in on problems and solutions without wasting time considering alternatives. For these nurses, the knowledge imbedded in practice starts to become visible.

The Dreyfus educational model allowed Benner to segregate and rank anecdotes about excellent practice among nurses. An important finding was that the nursing process worked better at lower levels of expertise than at higher ones. This may account for its popularity in schools (it provides a structure for the learner) and for the fact that many experienced, practicing nurses seem to ignore it.

Benner found the need for a rigidly controlled system (and the nursing process/nursing diagnosis system is just that) was greatest for the novice or advanced beginner, but that such high control actually impaired the work of the expert nurse: "If experts are made to attend to the particulars or to a formal model or rule, then performance actually deteriorates." (Benner, 1984, p. 37)

THEORY BUILDING WITH THE NURSING PROCESS

The nursing process alone is simply a theory strand, not a complete theory. The attempt to build a comprehensive theory around it can be seen in two movements: (1) the attempt to use the nursing process in conjunction with other theories that lack a process element, and (2) the effort to taxonomize nursing diagnoses and interventions as complementary content pieces.

Capers and Kelly (1987, p. 19) illustrate the first tactic when they appended the nursing process to Neuman's (1980) theory. Neuman's theory, like the nursing process, is logistic and reductionist, so combining these two systems is possible. In the adaptation made here, the authors used Neuman's organizing categories of psychological, physiologic, developmental, sociocultural, and spiritual as the content items (diagnostic categories) to which the nursing process was applied.

One can envision a similar appending of nursing process to Johnson's (1980) content categories (human behavioral systems). One could *not* use the same tactic on Roy's (1980) theory, on the other hand, even though she has a logistic system, because she has developed her own process element (stimulus–response manipulation). The introduction of the nursing process into this work would be a major theory alteration. (Of course, some are doing just that in practice and in educational programs.)

The more common tactic is not to link nursing process with an extant theory but to produce new content to accommodate it. Loomis and Wood (1983) gave an example of such a constructed theory. Their *process* element (called *clinical decision making*) is a formulation of the nursing process with elements of data collecting, diagnosing, planning, treating, and evaluating. In their model, a second set of interfacing components identifies actual or potential health problems. This category includes developmental life changes, acute health deviation, chronic health deviation, and cultural/environmental stressors. These theory elements can best be interpreted as *context* elements, that is, circumstances under which nursing occurs. A final set of factors identifies human responses, including physical, emotional, cognitive, familial, social, and cultural. This set represents *content* items.

The Loomis and Wood model illustrates a nursing theory constructed by combining nursing process with other elements, in this case, health problems and human responses. A more common tactic is to link nursing process with nursing diagnoses.

Nursing Diagnosis and Intervention

Although nursing diagnosis has wide acceptance in nursing, there has never been consensus on what it means. Yet the work on nursing diagnosis is one of the few successful group endeavors in theory building. Gebbie and Lavin (1975) reported on the initial 1973 work of the First National Conference on the Classification of Nursing Diagnoses. As one might expect, the first group effort produced as much confusion as light. From the start, there were complaints about many of the items labeled as diagnoses. The same year that the report was published, Gebbie (1975) clarified the definition of a nursing diagnosis as follows:

> A nursing diagnosis is a label for a condition most clearly identified by nurses, and amenable to treatment using the range of nursing skills. It remains a nursing diagnosis even if made by another; for example, "sensory deprivation" would seem to many to be a nursing rather than a medical diagnosis. . . .
> . . . what is a diagnosis in one discipline may be a sign of a different diagnosis in another. For example, "fracture of femur" is a medical diagnosis. "Limitation of mobility" is accepted by many as a nursing diagnosis (p. 69).

The diagnoses determined by that First National Conference on the Classification of Nursing Diagnoses represented many different sorts of items from soup to nuts. They included the following five items:

1. states of being experienced by the patient—and possibly inferred by the nurse (e.g., pain, anxiety, confusion)
2. physiologic deviations from the norm (e.g., irregular bowel function, impaired mobility)

3. patient behaviors perceived as problematic by the nurse (e.g., noncompliance, manipulation)
4. altered relationships by the patient, on which value judgments have been placed by the nurse (e.g., alteration in faith in God, altered relations with self and others)
5. reactions of another party (e.g., significant other's adjustment to patient's illness; Gebbie & Lavin, 1975, pp. 62–112).

Work on nursing diagnosis is still underway almost 20 years later, now carried on by individuals and in group activity by the North American Nursing Diagnosis Association (NANDA). NANDA (1989) has released a taxonomy of diagnoses, probably the most used taxonomy today. Even though this group has made refinements in what constitutes a diagnosis, the taxonomy still has its critics—as does the notion of nursing diagnosis itself.

Porter (1986) has asserted that NANDA has subordinated the task of creating a taxonomy to politics:

> These purposes [for having a taxonomy] are all related to promoting the unique identity of the nursing profession; while this is a commendable aim, it is quite different from the traditional purpose of taxonomic development (p. 136).

She has reminded us that taxonomies are used to explain why an object has various propertics similar to and different from others in its class. This precludes the NANDA attempts to force nursing diagnoses into a conceptual framework consisting of categories that are not mutually exclusive or jointly exhaustive.

Although Porter has addressed the NANDA work in its specifics, Turkoski (1988) has pointed out confusions that apply more generally. Her concerns have revolved around the nature of a nursing diagnosis, and she has identified disagreements on many poles: whether a nursing diagnosis can also be a medical diagnosis, whether a nursing diagnosis is different from a nursing assessment, and whether individual items qualify in various taxonomies.

P. H. Mitchell, Gallucci, and Fought (1991) have called for a new organization for diagnoses; suggesting the following four human responses: (1) behavioral, (2) experiential, (3) pathophysiologic, and (4) physiologic (p. 154). They are not the only critics who would change the work being done on the diagnosis element. But, on the whole, disagreements are fewer these days, and categories—at least those evolved by NANDA—have been refined and extended.

Just as we found authors who applied the nursing process to theories that lacked a process element, so we find authors trying to

link the notion of nursing diagnosis to already existing theories. See
Jenny (1989) for an attempt at reconciling the NANDA classification
with Orem's (1985) (process) concept of self-care. For work on diagnosis done by individuals, see, for example, diagnostic taxonomies by
Doenges and Moorhouse (1988), Gordon (1982), Kim, McFarland,
and McLane (1984), and Carpenito (1984).

A comprehensive taxonomy of nursing diagnoses is a perfect
fit with the nursing process—a process in search of content. Now
attention is turning to development of taxonomies for nursing interventions. It is interesting that no one is doing major work on taxonomies for prognoses or goal setting—categories that logically fit between diagnosis and intervention. Somehow these two steps of the
nursing process have never received much attention and are often
hidden intellectual steps unrecognized even by the nurses who perform them.

The work of Bulechek and McCloskey (1987) heralded serious
work on the intervention phase. Their early work specified nursing
interventions that were separate from physicians' orders, activities
that fell within the independent role of nursing. They included actions such as relaxation training, counseling, values clarification,
music therapy, and exercise programs among others.

Their work at the University of Iowa has now grown beyond the
esoteric interventions of holistic nursing into an endeavor to truly
capture all the normal interventions the constitute the work of nursing. This endeavor, indeed, is conceived as part of the effort to create
a nursing minimum data set (Werley & Lang, 1988). The final set
is envisioned as containing nursing diagnoses, interventions, and
patient outcomes.

Bulechek and McCloskey (1992) have differentiated between diagnoses and interventions by saying that diagnoses represent a client
behavior or status, whereas interventions describe a nurse behavior
(p. 290). Their labels consist of three words or fewer, such as *bleeding
reduction: nasal* or *cardiac care: acute* (pp. 293–294). Their work
in creating labels is extensive, with more than 3000 nursing activities
considered and more than 400 resultant labels (p. 291).

What the University of Iowa group is attempting to do with interventions has already been organized for nurses in home health care
(Saba et al., 1991). Saba et al. developed a computerized classification
system in relation to services for Medicare patients. They used 80,000
textual descriptions as a data source, making the system one of the
most comprehensive designs yet to surface.

No theory is without real limitations, and that is certainly true
of the nursing process/diagnosis/intervention model. Although the
nursing process steps are easily learned and used by inexperienced

nurses, the nursing diagnoses are so numerous that they make application a trial. Although the taxonomies of nursing interventions are just coming on the scene and not yet in common use, one can anticipate that the extensive number of labels will present the same problems as do the long lists of diagnoses. The question is whether such a complex system can have a major impact on practice. The argument against this complaint is that a similar system of diagnostic classification has worked effectively in medicine for years. Yet there is a difference in the two applications. Physicians use an operational system (differential diagnosis) rather than a logistic schema. They feel no need to consider the whole list of possibilities; they select those that suit their purposes and deal with them alone. Physicians also do not feel a need to refer to the official codes when diagnosing and treating patients. Nurses, in contrast, are concerned with their lists and the sorts of items composing those lists. They tend to view the lists of diagnoses as documents to use in relation to client work, not as a system primarily for statistical and taxonomic (as opposed to clinical) purposes.

Weber (1991), aware of the criticisms against nursing diagnosis, claimed that the fault lies in the application, not in the diagnoses themselves. She outlined a step-by-step approach designed to make the system useable. She also reminded us that the diagnostic system is still in its infancy, and we should not expect all glitches to disappear over night.

Geissler (1991) has also criticized the work of NANDA, claiming it is culture bound when viewed from a transcultural nursing perspective. She identified the following three flaws in the work, which:

1. assumes the patient is "wrong" and the provider is "right"
2. generalizes or stereotypes behaviors
3. mislabels the etiologic basis of a patient's problem as cultural without recognizing other potentially more relevant variables (p. 203).

G. J. Mitchell (1991) has reminded us that the system cannot escape the dangers of labeling and stereotyping—tactics that nurses have decried when others have used them. Scahill (1991) has added a concern that the separate list of nursing diagnoses may put nurses at risk of isolation in multidisciplinary settings such as psychiatry. The use of NANDA diagnostic labels has always been especially tricky in psychiatry. For a sense of these complexities, see Vincent and Coler's (1990) attempt to bridge the gap between NANDA efforts and the classification work of the ANA Task Force on the Classification of Phenomena in Psychiatric-Mental Health Nursing.

Nevertheless, because the system of nursing diagnosis is designed for reaching consensus (an acceptable level of agreement among users) its final success or failure will be judged on that basis. So far, the results are mixed. In a study by Levin, Krainovitch, Bahrenburg, and Mitchell (1989), for example, five out of six tested diagnoses (NANDA list) reached acceptable levels of agreement among users. In contrast, Andersen and Briggs (1988) found nurses lacked proficiency in formulating valid nursing diagnoses (p. 144). The Dennison and Keeling (1989) study of one NANDA category—knowledge deficit—found serious problems with the concept. These are only three of many studies, and, so far, there is no consensus on content validity or reliability of the labels.

PROBLEM-ORIENTED NURSING

Like the nursing process, problem-oriented nursing is only a partial theory. Alone, it lacks context and content. Just as the nursing process is commonly linked to one or another content item, so problem-oriented nursing comprises a method (problem solving) that may be linked to various patient or nursing problems (content). Problem-oriented nursing is a model that competes with the nursing process in practice. Originating with Dewey (1938) and applied early in educational theory, problem solving was described as the problematic method in Chapter 10. The reader may wish to review that chapter before proceeding. To differentiate the problem-solving structure from that of the nursing process, a brief comparison on four points follows:

1. Problem solving occurs when a nurse meets an obstacle—situational or intellectual—that starts her on a search for more information. The nursing process, on the other hand, starts with assessment simply because a person has been labeled *patient*. There is no waiting for an obstacle to appear.
2. Problem solving is less formal than the nursing process. There is much back and forth between the problem as tentatively cast and the environment where explanations and solutions are sought. As the problem is redefined and delimited, the environment that applies to the case itself shifts. The nursing process, in contrast, follows an invariant sequence in which the diagnosis flows from the assessment data, and each subsequent step follows from the preceding one. This invariable sequence has no back-and-forth adjustment. Diagnoses, for example, are derived from assessments; nursing prescriptions are derived from goals set.

3. Problem solving has as its aim defining the situation. This is
more important in one sense than the solution because the
character of the problem will determine the arena of and the
characteristics of the solution sought. When achieved, the
right solution is the one that gets rid of the problem. Problem
solving aims to eliminate the obstacle, and there may be
diverse ways to do so. The nursing process, in contrast, does
not aim to get rid of anything. Instead, it sets a specific goal
(e.g., to have the patient walk with a four-point gait by the
third week with adequate muscle strength for crutch
management). Instead of seeking a resolution, the nursing
process seeks to achieve one or more identified and specified
goals.
4. Problem solving is highly personal in that the nurse initiates
the process because something bothers her. If she is not
bothered by a situation (e.g., a patient's slowed speech), then
there is not any problem to be solved. The problem only exists
when she recognizes it—however tentatively she may define
it. The nursing process, on the other hand, is abstracted from
the personal. If the rules and processes are accurately
followed, any two nurses should draw the same conclusions,
set the same goals, select like interventions.

Take as a final illustration a comparison of how assessment might
occur in the two contrasting systems. In the nursing process, assessment would be complete, from head to toe—probably working from
a highly structured format. The process would be applied no matter
what the patient's complaints or status.

In problem solving, in contrast, the nurse would focus on the
patient's problem, and the assessments she would perform would be
those that related to the problem. For example, if the problem were
a fractured metacarpal incurred in a minor accident, the nurse would
be unlikely to perform a pelvic examination—and even more unlikely
to tolerate a list that said she should examine "everything."

Although problem solving was touted as *the* nursing method at
one time in nursing, it was shortly superseded in popularity by the
nursing process (proving the futility of advocating any one method
as an absolute standard). The form in which problem solving retains
some popularity is the Weed (1978) or so-called problem-oriented
system of charting. It has been adapted and adopted by many institutions. In these organizations, nurses, physicians, or both chart according to the problems evinced by the patient. Often nursing notes must
be categorized according to patient problems. The structure forces
the nurse to think in a problem-solving modality; she cannot chart

except as her efforts relate to the resolution of one or another perceived problem.

As with the nursing process, the content to be used in problem-oriented nursing has been the subject of much debate. In a pure problematic version, there are no constrictions on what counts as a problem. The nurse is the one to identify the problem; its ultimate delineation is unique and depends on her enquiry processes.

Sometimes the problem-oriented system is modified by supplying the nurse with a list of "appropriate problems" from which to select. This tactic shifts the system from a problematic format to an operational or logistic one, not unlike the use of nursing diagnosis lists. Some authorities advocate a shared list of problems between medicine and nursing; others advocate a separate and distinct list of nursing problems. In any case, once the so-called problems have already been defined, prescribed, and labeled, one is no longer actually using the problem-solving method. The crux of a problematic method is determining the unique problem.

Just as advocates of nursing process debate over the proper form for nursing diagnoses, so those recommending problem solving argue over what type of problem qualifies. Some like the perspective of *nursing* problems, that is, problems for the nurse such as fluid and electrolyte imbalance, cyanosis, failure to comply with a nursing regimen. Others select *patient* problems, for example, pain, anxiety, or immobility, in other words, problems directly perceived by patients.

BLENDING PROBLEM SOLVING AND
THE NURSING PROCESS

Not all authors make the discrimination between problem solving and the nursing process that this book offers. Nevertheless, I think mixing these modalities is confusing and makes caring for patients (and thinking about their needs) more difficult for nurses. Consider, for example, the nurse who must fill out a nursing care plan based on the nursing process, yet simultaneously chart in accordance with a problem-oriented schema. Surely she will have difficulty determining which modality directs her nursing behavior. See McHugh (1986) for a careful analysis of this issue from the perspective of what the nursing process is and is not.

Other authors see problem solving and the nursing process as perfectly compatible systems. For example, LaMonica (1979) has equated nursing diagnoses in one system with problems in the other. She found other parallelisms between the two systems, equating both nursing process and problem-oriented recording with the scientific method (p. 318). Essentially, she found their differences more a matter of form than substance. LaMonica is not alone in this interpretation; many other nurses treat the two systems as identical.

SUMMARY

Many theory threads are used in today's practice of nursing. These threads compose partial theories of nursing. Some are being further developed with the aim of producing a comprehensive theory. Others are conjoined with diverse theory strands, participating in many different theories (complete or partial). At present, the two most popular process threads are nursing process and problem solving. But the nursing process far exceeds problem-oriented nursing in popularity.

REFERENCES

Andersen, J. E., & Briggs, L. L. (1988). Nursing diagnosis: A study of quality and supportive evidence. *Image, 3,* 141–144.

Benner, P. (1984). *From novice to expert: Excellence and power in clinical nursing practice.* Menlo Park, CA: Addison-Wesley.

Bulechek, G. M., & McCloskey, J. C. (1987). Nursing interventions: What they are and how to choose them. *Holistic Nursing Practice, 3,* 36–44.

Bulechek, G. M., & McCloskey, J. C. (1992). Defining and validating nursing intervention. *Nursing Clinics of North America, 2,* 289–299.

Capers, C. F., & Kelly, R. (1987). Neuman nursing process: A model of holistic care. *Holistic Nursing Practice, 3,* 19–26.

Carpenito, L. J. (1984). *Handbook of nursing diagnosis.* Philadelphia: J. B. Lippincott.

Dennison, P. D., & Keeling, A. W. (1989). Clinical support for eliminating the nursing diagnosis of knowledge deficit. *Image, 3,* 142–144.

Dewey, J. (1938). *Logic: The theory of inquiry.* New York: Henry Holt.

Doenges, M. E., & Moorhouse, M. F. (1988). *Nurse's pocket guide: Nursing diagnosis with interventions* (2nd ed.). Philadelphia: F. A. Davis.

Dreyfus, S. E., & Dreyfus, H. L. (undated). *A five-stage model of the mental activities involved in directed skill acquisition* (unpublished report, United States Air Force Office of Scientific Research, Contract No. F49620-79-C-0063). Berkeley: University of California.

Gebbie, K. M. (1975). Development of a taxonomy of nursing diagnosis. In J. B. Walter, G. P. Pardee, & D. M. Molbo (Eds.), *Dynamics of problem oriented approaches: Patient care and documentation* (pp. 65–76). New York: J. B. Lippincott.

Gebbie, K. M., & Lavin, M. A. (Eds.). (1975). *Proceedings of the first national conference: Classification of nursing diagnoses.* St. Louis, MO: C. V. Mosby.

Geissler, E. M. (1991). Transcultural nursing and nursing diagnoses. *Nursing & Health Care, 4,* 109–192, 203.

Gordon, M. (1982). *Manual of nursing diagnosis.* New York: McGraw-Hill.

Henderson, V. (1987). Nursing process—A critique. *Holistic Nursing Practice, 3,* 7–18.

Jenny, J. (1989). Classifying nursing diagnoses: A self-care approach. *Nursing & Health Care, 2,* 83–88.

Johnson, D. E. (1980). The behavioral system model for nursing. In J. P. Riehl & C. Roy (Eds.), *Conceptual models for nursing practice* (2nd ed., pp. 207–216). New York: Appleton-Century-Crofts.

Kim, M. J., McFarland, G. K., & McLane, A. M. (Eds.). (1984). *Pocket guide to nursing diagnoses.* St. Louis, MO: C. V. Mosby.

Kobert, L., & Folan, M. (1990). Coming of age in nursing: Rethinking the philosophies behind holism and nursing process. *Nursing & Health Care, 6,* 308–312.

LaMonica, E. L. (1979). *The nursing process: A humanistic approach.* Menlo Park, CA: Addison-Wesley.

Levin, R. F., Krainovitch, B. C., Bahrenburg, E., & Mitchell, C. A. (1989). Diagnostic content validity of nursing diagnosis. *Image, 1,* 40–44.

Loomis, M. E., & Wood, D. J. (1983). Cure: The potential outcome of nursing care. *Image, 1,* 4–7.

McHugh, M. (1986). Nursing process: Musings on the method. *Holistic Nursing Practice, 1,* 21–28.

Mitchell, G. J. (1991). Nursing diagnosis: An ethical analysis. *Image, 2,* 99–103.

Mitchell, P. H., Gallucci, B., & Fought, S. G. (1991). Perspectives on human response to health and illness. *Nursing Outlook, 4,* 154–157.

Neuman, B. (1980). The Betty Neuman health-care systems model: A total person approach to patient problems. In J. P. Riehl & C. Roy (Eds.), *Conceptual models for nursing practice* (2nd ed., pp. 119–134). New York: Appleton-Century-Crofts.

North American Nursing Diagnosis Association. (1989). *Taxonomy I revised—1989: With official diagnostic categories.* St. Louis, MO: Author.

Roy, C. (1980). The Roy adaptation model. In J. P. Riehl & C. Roy (Eds.), *Conceptual models for nursing practice* (2nd ed., pp. 179–188). New York: Appleton-Century-Crofts.

Porter, E. J. (1986). Critical analysis of NANDA nursing diagnosis taxonomy I. *Image, 4,* 136–139.

Orem, D. E. (1985). *Nursing: Concepts of practice* (3rd ed.). New York: McGraw-Hill.

Saba, V. K., O'Hare, P. A., Zuckerman, A. E., Boondas, J., Levine, E., & Oatway, D. M. (1991). A nursing intervention taxonomy for home health care. *Nursing & Health Care, 6,* 296–299.

Scahill, L. (1991). Nursing diagnosis vs. goal-oriented treatment planning in inpatient child psychiatry. *Image, 2,* 95–97.

Turkoski, B. B. (1988). Nursing diagnosis in print, 1950–1985. *Nursing Outlook, 4,* 142–144.

Vincent, K. G., & Coler, M. S. (1990). A unified nursing diagnostic model. *Image, 2,* 93–95.

Weber, G. (1991). Making nursing diagnosis work for you and your client: A step-by-step approach. *Nursing & Health Care, 8,* 424–430.

Weed, L. (1978). *Medical records, medical education, and patient care.* Cleveland, OH: Press of Case Western Reserve University.

Werley, H. H., & Lang, N. M. (Eds.). (1988). *Identification of the nursing minimum data set.* New York: Springer.

12 Systems Models in Nursing Theory

SYSTEMS VERSUS SYSTEMATIC

Many nurse theorists claim to have a systems approach to nursing theory. If fact, some do and some do not. It is important to understand what writers mean by *systems*, because different writers mean different things. For some the meaning may be so casual as to mean systematic. Indeed, we assume that a good theory in any format would be systematic rather than chaotic. Therefore, to use the term *systems* in this fashion trivializes it.

For our purposes, we will use the term *systems model* to apply to a theory that treats its subject matter as consisting of component parts and their interrelationships. In the systems approach, the focus is on the discrete parts and their interrelationships, which make up and describe the whole (i.e., the system). The system (the whole) is no more than the sum of its parts and their relationships.

If this sounds familiar, it is because a logistic pattern of thought is the backbone of a systems model. Systems, then, are tightly structured designs with intentional application of logistic patterns of thought. Systems models are those in which the pattern of relationships among parts is highly prescribed. The nursing process discussed in Chapter 11 would qualify as a systems model; the problem-solving model, obviously, would not.

Keep in mind that the subject matter addressed by a theory is not what characterizes a system. The subject matters of nursing systems include man as a system (Johnson, 1980; Neuman, 1980; Roy, 1980), the patient–nurse interaction system (King, 1981), larger systems such as communities or societies (also King, 1981), and organizations such as health care systems (Arndt & Huckabay, 1975).

Barbara J. Stevens Barnum: NURSING THEORY:
ANALYSIS, APPLICATION, EVALUATION, FOURTH EDITION.
© 1994, 1990, 1984, 1979 J.B. Lippincott.

For any given subject matter (e.g., man as a system), there can be major differences from theorist to theorist. The components of Johnson's (1980) man-system are behavioral subsystems (such as aggression, affiliation, achievement), whereas Roy's (1980) components of the man-system are adaptation modes: physiologic, self-concept, role function, and interdependence relations. One cannot assume that the subject matter alone is a clue as to whether a theory is a systems model.

METHODOLOGY

Whatever their subject matter, systems-oriented theorists focus on methodology by discussing their subject matter in ways that

- differentiate the *system* from its environment (i.e., identify boundary lines or events)
- describe input from the environment into the system as well as output from the system back to the environment (an open system model as opposed to a closed system that does not interact across its boundaries)
- identify the energy or motivation of the system (i.e., what makes the system work, keep going, or, in its absence, slow down and stop)
- consider system equilibrium, or what keeps the system in balance, stable, within acceptable limits (as opposed to developmental changes in which the subject matter changes, evolves, takes on new goals, or radically alters its structures)
- identify the goals toward which the system strives and that dictate the nature of what happens in the system
- describe the thruput or central processing (what the system does to the input), usually in terms of a finite series of sequential acts or events over time
- identify feedback or cybernetic components, allowing output and goal to be compared, and giving information that is used in system adjustment
- explain the given system, itself, as consisting of smaller subsystems or explain the system as itself being a subsystem of a larger system.

Different theorists may stress different aspects of the systems approach, while still maintaining the general design. For example, one theorist may focus on the system-environment boundary events (e.g., human response to environmental stressors); a second theorist may focus on the specific nature of the thruput (structure of the central processing). A third theorist may focus on the process or movement of raw materials (input) through the system to their output as finished product, whereas a fourth theorist may focus on cybernetic events (e.g., system adjustments in light of output).

Theories Stressing Boundary Events

Theories stressing boundary events focus on intake or exchange. For example, if man is the system under consideration, one might focus on biologic intake (food, oxygen, microbes) or on biologic exchange (the human ecology approach). The same exchange approach might be used in relation to the social environment to examine reciprocal or unequal exchanges of affect. Some ecofeminist theories might be coined in terms of social exchange.

Instead of looking at the content of the materials entering or leaving the system, some theories are concerned primarily with the energy flow. Man, for example, may be seen as taking more energy from the environment than he returns to it, using the energy for growth (*negentropy*). Notice that a theory such as this might use a term (energy) as do Newman (1986) and Rogers (1990), but this does not mean Newman's and Rogers's theories are systems models. They are not; they are developmental models with dialectic thought structures.

Other systems theories are concerned with entry criteria. For example, a systems model might be concerned with what constitutes a nursing act and what does not. Systems models tend to be clear and crisp about their components. In this case, precise decision rules would determine what examples of nurse behavior qualify for processing in the system.

Theories Stressing the Structure of the Thruput

The theorist who focuses on the thruput examines the system from the perspective of structure. Thruput often is reflected in flowcharts (Figure 12–1). Such a chart shows what happens to the materials entering the system. The thruput segment is sometimes called the *black box* if its processes are as yet not fully understood. In Johnson's (1980) theory, for example, one might say that the relationships among her subsystems of behavior are yet to be fully explored and described. The exact relationship of achievement behavior to affiliative behavior, for example, has yet to be determined. Yet in principle, she would admit that these interactions of subcomponents do occur.

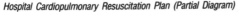

Hospital Cardiopulmonary Resuscitation Plan (Partial Diagram)

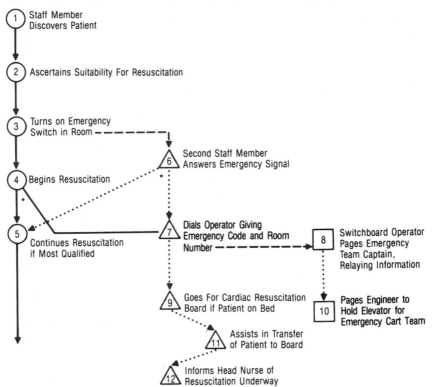

Figure 12–1. *Thruput component of a systems model, using flow charts to illustrate partial hospital cardiopulmonary resuscitation plan. *, path choice point.*

Theories Stressing Processes of the System

The theorist who focuses on process rather than structure is likely to use a model such as Figure 12–2. Applying this model to the patient as input, one arrives at Figure 12–3. Note that, in this example, the nursing organization, rather than the patient, is the system.

Theories Stressing Cybernetics

Another focus, on the cybernetic system, concentrates on the feedback loop as illustrated in Figure 12–4. Note that the feedback loop has three functions: (1) production of data concerning system output, (2) comparison of data to preestablished goals, and (3) adjustment of the system for better goal achievement. Typically, the adjustment occurs in the thruput, but regulation is sometimes accom-

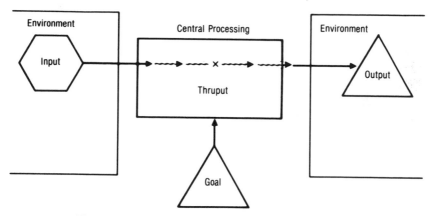

Figure 12–2. *Basic systems model (process type).*

plished through change in input or alteration of the goals themselves.

A specific nursing goal and its measurement are illustrated in Figure 12–5. In this example, the cybernetic loop becomes the model for quality control of patient care. Patient outcomes are compared with patient care standards, and related nursing acts (thruput) will be adjusted accordingly.

The Joint Commission on the Accreditation of Health Care Organizations has shifted its perspective from examining input (structure) and thruput (process) to a closer look at the cybernetic loop, namely a concern with output. In a sense, this is a welcome change because outcomes are the whole point of health care. The shift in focus by the accrediting agency, however, has required major shifts in record

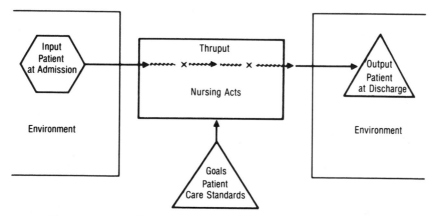

Figure 12—3. *Basic systems model of nursing care delivery.*

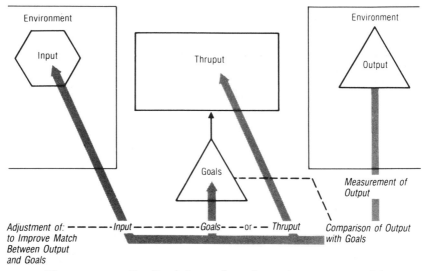

Figure 12–4. Feedback loop of a cybernetic systems model.

keeping and quality assurance plans in institutions across the United States. In a sense, the shift to the cybernetic aspect of care delivery completes an inevitable cycle that could have been predicted. Indeed, comparing the new accrediting system to the older process reveals how much diversity can occur—all within a systems ideology.

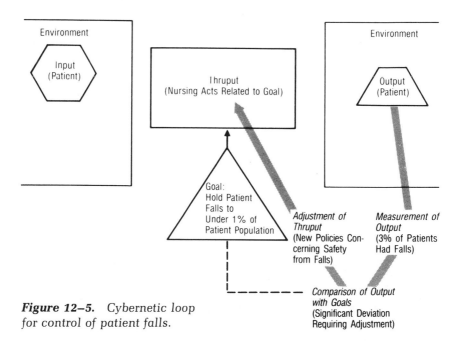

Figure 12–5. Cybernetic loop for control of patient falls.

MISLEADING USES OF SYSTEMS TERMINOLOGY

We have already discussed the confusing use of the term *systems* to cover every instance of systematic thought. A second and common error is the application of the systems label to dialectic constructs in which the whole is more than the sum of its parts, and, indeed, when it is the whole that gives meaning to the parts. For example, if one were to describe a nursing service organization (subject matter) as having a certain organizational *personality*, and furthermore, if one stated that this organizational personality caused head nurses to act in a particular way, then one is *not* talking in terms of a logistic system. In this example, the "system" is dialectic because characteristics of the whole account for characteristics of the part.

A dialectic model focuses on the constellation created by the parts, not on the parts themselves. When a part is singled out for attention, it is explained by virtue of the constellation, that is, what happens to the part is seen as occurring because of its relation to the whole. A person filling the scapegoat role in a family is an example of a part (person) explained in relation to the whole (family), not in terms of that person's discrete and separate relations with other individuals in the family.

It is not unusual to see theories misclassified in nursing texts. For example, in Roy's (1980) edited work, Rogers's (1990) theory is inappropriately listed as a systems model. Rogers's theory is clearly dialectic, not logistic. Many authors differentiate logistic and dialectic models into systems and developmental models, respectively. Developmental models differ from systems models in that their goals, components, and structures are capable of and predisposed to change, usually toward ever greater levels of complexity, with qualitative changes in nature, not merely quantitative addition of new parts. Where Maslow's (1954) hierarchy of needs is seen as describing emerging stages of man, then emergence of a qualitatively different need would be developmental, an instance in which the entity itself was changed radically.

A systems model typically does not evolve and develop, but it can grow more complex by adding new components. When a new component is added, it is simply integrated with the system components already described.

Because most dialectic models also are developmental, the division between systems models and developmental models usually serves to differentiate logistic and dialectic systems. Chrisman and Fowler (1980), however, have presented a model (the systems-developmental stress model) that confounds the difference between systems and developmental models, viewing man developmentally from birth to death, but claiming that in any given slice of time, he can be viewed as consisting of interlocking biologic, social, and personal systems. Although verbal support is given to the developmental aspect, the theory itself operates on a logistic method. As with many logistic models that take man as the subject matter, this model's input is a set of stressors and its focus is the cybernetic adaptation of the system.

Another misleading use of systems terms occurs when an entity is described by a systems model (as parts and relationships), but its components and relationships do not really represent thruput processes. Take, for example, Arndt and Huckabay's (1975) model of nursing administration. Within what is claimed to be a systems model, their peculiar pattern of components and relationships is illustrated in Figure 12–6.

Use of diagrams and flowcharts is a common and useful way to indicate relations in a systems model. Note, however, that the Arndt and Huckabay diagram does not really represent a sequential flow of events. If one carefully reads the verbs that link components, it is apparent that Component B is an output term, Component C a goal term, Component D a thruput step, and Component E is probably a side effect.

The two-directional arrows of this model further confound the reader because they eliminate sequence and introduce confusion. For example, that Component A creates Component B would seem

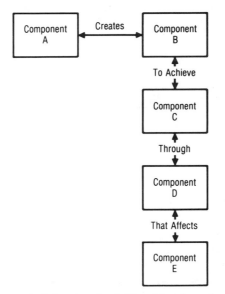

Figure 12–6. *Segment of structural relationships, based on model by Arndt and Huckabay.*

to contradict that Component B creates A, a statement one can make equally well according to the arrows in this diagram. Although co-creation is no problem in a developmental model—see Parse (1981), for example—it just does not fit in a systems model. Hence, one distraction in analyzing theory is the application of systems-like flowcharts to components and relationships that actually do not express a system.

In contrast, the systems model of the nursing process in Gordon's (1982) book (on the inside front cover) is an accurate use of systems, with each step leading the next. Gordon has elaborated 14 direct steps, formalizing some of the actions that occur unrecognized in shorter versions of the nursing process. In addition, her model has interim decision exit points (a perfectly legitimate logistic tactic) and a feedback loop.

A final problem in systems models is the overcomplex model that specifies components and relationships too numerous to conceptualize. The net effect of such specificity is that the reader (let alone the theorist) is unable to calculate the effect of a given system manipulation. Neuman's (1980) model, interrelating more than 35 variables, typifies this pattern of complexity. Although such a model may be a legitimate logistic method, it fails the test for parsimony. As mentioned in Chapter 11, this is a flaw in the elaborate nursing process/diagnosis/intervention model.

Of course, in a day of extending and expanding computerization programming, it is possible to build highly complex systems with interacting and interdependent parts that defy human intuitive comprehension. The computerization of nursing diagnoses and interventions has proven this point. For theories with massive numbers of components, it may be that the best one can hope for is to intuitively grasp the principle by which the system functions and let the computer calculate the effects of interface changes.

COMPUTERIZATION AND SYSTEMS MODELS

Today, much of the major growth in nursing involves the development of what is termed *nursing informatics,* namely the growth and expansion in use of computerization in nursing. The ways in which computers are applied to nursing will help shape tomorrow's nursing theories. Already we have seen the development of the nursing process/diagnosis/intervention model. Other designs may follow in the future.

There is no question that computer systems will affect our future. Yet computers, by necessity, function in patterns of logistic (linear) relationships or in branching logic (an operational variation). It is perhaps ironic that these systems are developing side by side with a new thrust toward holistic theories antithetical to this mode of thought. Will nursing find a way to accommodate these two theory developments simultaneously? With the exception of nursing process/diagnosis/intervention, nursing systems theories have declined in popularity. The reader with a strong interest in systems design might do well to read about nursing informatics with her "theory-colored glasses" on. Theories developing in the systems design are likely to rely heavily on computer technology, following software and hardware capabilities. True, there is some talk of computers so sophisticated that they can escape their highly prescribed program formats—a computer designed to enhance its own learning potential, for example. But it is likely to be a long time before computers can replicate the changing visions of holistic nursing theory.

SUMMARY

The use of systems terminology in relation to nursing theories requires close scrutiny. Writers mean different things by the term *system*. It would be simpler if the systems label were reserved for logistic systems to avoid this confusion. The following three misleading uses of systems were identified as consonant with this description:

1. the use of systems to describe *any* systematic work
2. the use of systems to describe dialectic or developmental constellations
3. the application of flowcharts and diagrams that inaccurately appear to be logistic to describe nonlogistic theories.

Furthermore, even a legitimate systems model may be problematic in directing nursing practice if its variables are too numerous to grasp easily in the mind. On the other hand, good systems models, with their clear steps and controlled sequencing, are good learning tools for students. In addition, they allow for design of clear, precise research projects.

Systems models had a short flurry in nursing when they threatened to take over the domain of theory. At present, the strongest and most popular model is the nursing process/diagnosis/intervention system described in Chapter 11. In truth, this seems to be the only major systems contender among present nursing theories.

REFERENCES

Arndt, C., & Huckabay, L.M.D. (1975). *Nursing administration—Theory for practice with a systems approach*. St. Louis, MO: C.V. Mosby.
Chrisman, M. K., & Fowler, M. D. (1980). The systems-in-change model for

nursing practice. In J. P. Riehl & C. Roy (Eds.), *Conceptual models for nursing practice* (2nd ed., pp. 74–82). New York: Appleton-Century-Crofts.

Gordon, M. (1982). *Nursing diagnosis: Process and application.* New York: McGraw-Hill.

Johnson, D. E. (1980). The behavioral system model for nursing. In J. P. Riehl & C. Roy (Eds.), *Conceptual models for nursing practice* (2nd ed., pp. 207–216). New York: Appleton-Century-Crofts.

King, I. M. (1981). *A theory for nursing: Systems, concepts, process.* New York: Wiley.

Maslow, A. H. (1954). *Motivation and personality.* New York: Harper & Row.

Neuman, B. (1980). The Betty Neuman health-care systems model: A total person approach to patient problems. In J. P. Riehl & C. Roy (Eds.), *Conceptual models for nursing practice* (2nd ed., pp. 119–134). New York: Appleton-Century-Crofts.

Newman, M. A. (1986). *Health as expanding consciousness.* St. Louis, MO: C. V. Mosby.

Parse, R. R. (1981). *Man-living-health: A theory of nursing.* New York: Wiley.

Rogers, M. E. (1990). Nursing: Science of unitary, irreducible, human beings: Update 1990. In E.A.M. Barrett (Ed.), *Visions of Rogers' science-based nursing* (pp. 5–11). New York: National League for Nursing.

Roy, C. (1980). The Roy adaptation model. In J. P. Riehl & C. Roy (Eds.), *Conceptual models for nursing practice* (2nd ed., pp. 179–188). New York: Appleton-Century-Crofts.

BIBLIOGRAPHY

Bolwell, C. (1990). Evaluating computer-assisted-instruction. *Nursing & Health Care, 9,* 511–515.

Dediarian, A. K. (1990). The relationships among the subsystems of Johnson's behavioral system model. *Image, 4,* 219–225.

Fitzpatrick, J. J. (1988). How can we enhance nursing knowledge and practice? *Nursing & Health Care, 9,* 517–521.

Graves, J. R. (1989). The study of nursing informatics. *Image, 4,* 227–231.

Grubbs, J. (1980). An interpretation of the Johnson behavioral system model for nursing practice. In J. P Riehl & C. Roy (Eds.), *Conceptual models for nursing practice* (2nd ed., pp. 217–254). New York: Appleton-Century-Crofts.

Halloran, E. J. (1988). Computerized nurse assessments. *Nursing & Health Care, 9,* 497–499.

Heller, B. R., & Romano, C. A. (1988). Nursing informatics: The pathway to knowledge. *Nursing & Health Care, 9,* 483–484.

Jacox, A. (1974). Theory construction in nursing: An overview. *Nursing Research, 1,* 4–13.

McCormick, K. A. (1991). Future data needs for quality of care monitoring, DRG considerations, reimbursement and outcome measurement. *Image, 1,* 29–32.

Saba, V. K. (1988). Taming the computer jungle of NISs. *Nursing & Health Care, 9,* 487–491.

Scott, D, W., Oberst, M. T., & Dropkin, M. J. (1980). A stress-coping model. *Advances in Nursing Science, 1,* 9–24.

Sinclair, V. G. (1988). Database management: Solving information overload. *Nursing & Health Care, 9,* 493–495.

von Bertalanffy, L. (1968). *General systems theory: Foundations, applications* (rev. ed.). New York: George Braziller.

Weiler, K., & Rhodes, A. M. (1991). Legal methodology as nursing problem solving. *Image, 4,* 214–244.

13 Criteria for Evaluating Theories

THE NATURE OF JUDGMENT

Once a theory has been analyzed and classified, there remains the task of passing judgment on it. People often view the task of judgment from one of two positions:

1. Judgment is simply a matter of personal taste. Just as some persons prefer modern art to Renaissance art, some will prefer one theory to another. The merits of a given theory ultimately are matters of personal preference and taste.
2. There are certain clear criteria for judging nursing theories. Any reasonably intelligent and informed person, when applying these criteria, will arrive at similar judgments. Various theories are good, mediocre, or poor, and it is not only possible but reasonable to pass judgment on them.

In truth, there is some merit to both of these positions, because there are some evaluative criteria on which there is little consensus and others on which consensus is strong. Few nurses, for example, would debate the criterion of consistency, which calls for the use of terms in the same way throughout a theory work. On the other hand, there is little consensus on the criterion of scope. Some nurses judge a theory good if it covers a broad expanse of nursing practice and poor if its scope is a narrow slice of the nursing domain. Others would argue the opposite case.

This chapter looks at criteria of two sorts: those receiving general acceptance and those for which no consensus exists. Judgment of theories can be facilitated if internal and external criticisms are differentiated. Internal criticism deals with how theory components fit

Barbara J. Stevens Barnum: NURSING THEORY:
ANALYSIS, APPLICATION, EVALUATION, FOURTH EDITION.
© 1994, 1990, 1984, 1979 J.B. Lippincott.

with each other. It asks, Given the premises this theory assumes, does the reasoning logically follow? Do its pieces relate in a sensible pattern? Most people agree on judgments made using criteria for internal criticism; most members of a society use similar patterns of judgment regarding what are or are not logical relations.

External criticism deals with the way in which a theory relates to the extant world. It examines the premises a theory takes as the beginning points for its propositions (i.e., what is true about the world and nursing's function in it). Judgment here highly depends on individual preference—whether the given theory's view seems reasonable and reflects the world as perceived by the reader.

INTERNAL CRITICISM

Many criteria are applied in judging the internal construction of a theory—specifically, clarity, consistency, adequacy, and logical development. Usually there is agreement on the judgments made concerning these criteria. There is less agreement on the importance of a final criterion—the level of theory development.

Clarity

The criterion of clarity requires that a theory be presented in a way that can be easily understood by the reader. The issue of clarity is not to be confused with that of the simplicity or complexity of theory development, nor is it to be confused with the sequence in which the author presented material. The question is, Did she make sense of it?

In judging clarity, two sorts of meaning are given to terms. *Denotative* meaning is referential; it enables one to point out all the objects of a class, that is, all the objects to which a term refers. *Connotative* meaning, on the other hand, indicates what it is that denoted objects have in common. Connotation describes the characteristics of an object, giving the nuances of meaning and relaying the value bestowed.

Few authors have perfect clarity. Every author will slip now and then into a confusing sentence. But one must ask, How many sentences are meaningless? Do they preclude one's understanding of the theory? Are the basic terms themselves unclear? Are the terms clear as to both denotation and connotation? Are there obvious gaps in the theory that prevent the reader from linking parts of the theory with the subsequent aspects?

Consistency

The criterion of consistency can be applied in many different ways. We will examine inconsistencies in terms, interpretation, principle, and method. The simplest case involves definition of terms. Once a theorist has defined a term in a certain way, consistency requires that the term always be used in that way. Common errors occur when the theorist defines:

> nursing—as care of individuals or groups, but then goes on to discuss it only as it applies to care of the individual
>
> stress—as a vector acting on the body, but later includes bodily responses to the vector, thus combining cause and effect
>
> time—as the serial progression of clock minutes at one place and the perception of the time (the experience of duration) at another
>
> adaptation—as stimulus–response patterning, and later to mean psychological adjustment to a complex environmental change conceptualized in a Gestalt framework

The adaptation example represents more than a simple shift in the meaning of a term. Here, the fault includes a shift in the nature of the world being described. This shift in interpretation is a frequent fault in nursing theories. At one moment, a theory may view the world as consisting of physical entities that respond on the basis of neurohumoral rules, yet in the next instance, switch to a world view in which the major entities are, instead, noncorporeal constructs, such as spheres of influence, states of mind, or phases of development. The error does not relate to which is the *correct* interpretation of the external world (that would be an external criticism) but simply to the failure to be consistent in a world view.

Often the reader will miss an inconsistency of this sort because the author does not specifically describe the world to which her theory applies. The shift in the image of the world may be masked when the same theory terms are used throughout. For example, the continuous use of terms such as *adaptation* and *stress* may conceal the inconsistency of the world view. Such inconsistencies in interpretation often occur in theories that purport to synthesize elements from various disparate theory statements.

In addition to finding inconsistencies in the use of terms and in interpretation, the reader may find inconsistencies in principle. Suppose, for example, that a theory has reciprocal principles, one in the patient and one in the nursing act. Imagine that the principle explaining the patient is comprehensive (e.g., explaining man as some sort of holistic being). Suppose, on the other hand, that the principle of nursing action is entitative, relying on a stimulus–response explanation of behavior. Two such diverse principles would be inconsistent in a single theory; there is no logical way for the patient and nursing act to interrelate.

Similarly, one may find inconsistencies in relation to method. Often this occurs when trends in nursing dictate one method, whereas the author's own inclination follows a different path. The author may follow one method (her own) but give lip service to another method. In other cases, there may be fluctuations in method, making it impossible to classify.

Adequacy

A theory is adequate if it accounts for the subject matter with which it deals, however broad or limited the subject matter may be. A nursing theory is adequate if its prescriptions are extensive enough to cover the scope claimed by its author.

Rubin (1968), for example, presents an interesting theory of clinical nursing in which nursing is a helping technique "whereby the patient adjusts to, endures through, and usefully integrates the health problem situation in its many ramifications." (p. 210) In her conception, nursing care is an ever-changing interaction process, dependent on the moment-to-moment situation of the patient and his ability to cope with that situation. Situations, necessarily, are fluid in this model, and nursing is differentiated from other helping professions by its operation within the immediate present in relation to the patient's dependency needs. Some critics argue that this theory is appropriate for obstetrics (Rubin's specialty), but not for clinical nursing in general. The focus on immediacy, so say her critics, is built on the image of the patient in labor or in the midst of a major, immediate life change. The model, critics argue, fails to consider such elements as forward-looking health education or care of the patient with a chronic disease. Those who support the extended application of the theory claim that all notions of clinical nursing can be dealt with inside the model.

In some instances, a theory may so fit or misfit its purported scope that critics can easily agree whether it meets the criterion of adequacy. In other cases, such as Rubin's, the determination of match between theory and scope may call into question the reviewer's own conception of nursing. Hence, the criterion of adequacy sometimes reflects internal criticism, and other times, branches into external criticism.

Logical Development

The criterion of logical development requires that every conclusion set forth in a theory logically follow from the reasoning that has preceded it. Logical development demands that a conclusion be warranted, based on its premises. The study of logic reveals the structure of supported and unsupported arguments. Two examples are given, followed by the syllogistic form of each argument and an illustrative Venn diagram. These examples represent a deductive mode of reasoning in which a conclusion necessarily follows from its premises. Another mode of logical reasoning (induction) is discussed later. In Figure 13–1, the syllogistic form of the argument merely substitutes letters for terms, making the structure of the argument and its conclusion evident to the reader. The accompanying Venn diagram represents the interrelationship of the three terms of the argument. In the diagram, one blackens those portions of the representative circles not contained in the premises. Hence, because "All S is M" in this example, one blacks out the two segments of S that fall outside M. In looking at the second premise, two segments of P are similarly blackened. The remaining portions of the diagram reveal the error in the conclusion drawn. All remaining S is not P, so the argument is invalid.

Although the conclusion in the example may be patently illogical to the reader, the same pattern, given different terms, might lead the reader astray. Suppose, for example, that one substitutes *helping profession* for *communication*. The following argument results:

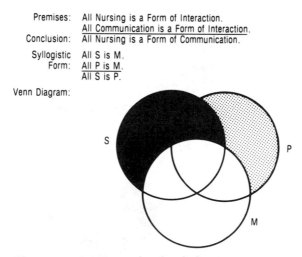

Premises:	All Nursing is a Form of Interaction.
	All Communication is a Form of Interaction.
Conclusion:	All Nursing is a Form of Communication.
Syllogistic Form:	All S is M.
	All P is M.
	All S is P.

Venn Diagram:

Figure 13–1. Example of a deductive argument.

All nursing is a form of interaction.
All helping professions are forms of interaction.
All nursing is a helping profession.

Note that the truth or falsity of the conclusion has nothing to do with the logical development of the argument. In this example, it may very well be true that nursing is a helping profession, but that conclusion cannot be drawn on the basis of these premises, even if the premises were assumed to be true. Logical development has to do with whether conclusions can be derived from given premises, not whether the given premises or conclusions are true. In Figure 13–2, the Venn diagram first blackens the inapplicable portions of the model. In addition, the second premise states that some portion of S must be M. An X is inserted in the unblackened segment, which meets this constraint, indicating that some of this segment *must* exist. For this argument, the syllogistic form can be supported (valid) because the extant segment of S falls within P, matching the conclusion drawn.

Obviously, many different forms of deductive argument can be postulated, and the Venn diagram is the traditional tool for determining the valid and invalid forms. In a deductive argument, one can say that a valid form is one in which the conclusion necessarily follows from the given premises. Furthermore, if the premises are true, then the conclusion necessarily is true.

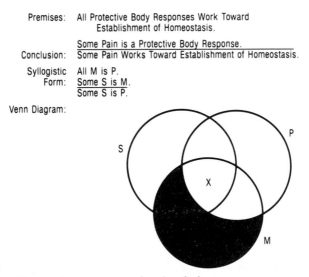

Premises: All Protective Body Responses Work Toward
            Establishment of Homeostasis.

            Some Pain is a Protective Body Response.
Conclusion: Some Pain Works Toward Establishment of Homeostasis.

Syllogistic   All M is P.
Form: Some S is M.
              Some S is P.

Venn Diagram:

Figure 13–2. *Example of a deductive argument.*

Inductive argument, in contrast, is based on probability rather than necessity. Induction depends on cases known, and the probability factor can always be changed by new, and contrary, cases. A typical inductive argument follows:

Morphine is a narcotic and relieves pain.
Codeine is a narcotic and relieves pain.
Heroin is a narcotic and relieves pain.
Therefore, all narcotics relieve pain.

As the reader knows, this inductive argument proves to be false, because some narcotics do not relieve pain. A single exception is all that is required to invalidate an inductive conclusion when the argument deals with absolutes. (It only takes one black swan to invalidate the assertion that all swans are white.) In the so-called soft sciences, inductive patterns may be tempered by frequency qualifiers or probability hedges (e.g., *most* patients prefer to know their diagnosis).

The reader who is unfamiliar with the logical syntax of inductive and deductive argument should invest in a basic work on logic such as Copi's (1982) work. This will enable the reader of theory to learn logical and illogical patterns of argument.

Do not confuse the logical development of an argument to its conclusion with the sequence used by the author in the written presentation of the argument. It is possible that the author may present the premises first, drawing the conclusions subsequently, or reveal the conclusions first, followed by the premises and argument from which they were derived. Logical development of a theory refers to the validity of its arguments, not to the sequence in the presentation.

Furthermore, logical development requires that a reader not have to supply missing links in an argument to reach (or agree with) a conclusion. Often the nurse reading a given theory supplies missing links, relying on her professional knowledge rather than on the theory as outlined. Indeed, the nurse may be unaware that she is filling in gaps.

In Chapter 11, we mentioned that some of the logical steps in the nursing process often were missing in written formulations. Take prognosis, for example. A prognosis influences nursing action in ways the nurse seldom thinks about. Imagine a patient with a severed spinal cord above the waist. Without recognizing that she is making a prognosis, the nurse will arrange her care around the thought that the patient will not walk again. The criterion of logical development, then, requires that a theory grow naturally from its premises, that its propositions follow from application of the rules of logic, and that any assertion or conclusion drawn flows reasonably from the groundwork laid for the assertion.

Level of Theory Development

Obviously, the ultimate aim of any theory is to reach the stage in which purposeful nursing interventions can be derived, leading to predictable patient outcomes—in other words, an explanatory theory with situation-producing capabilities. The level of theory development, however, is a function of historical time; every theory, at one time, begins with the descriptive naming of its elements.

It is possible that one theory, as yet in a descriptive phase, may hold more promise than another theory already in an explanatory phase of development. Therefore, a relatively low (early) level of theory development is not necessarily a drawback, certainly not in the same sense that lack of clarity, lack of consistency, or lack of logical development would be. Assessment of the level of theory development, of course, is an essential part of internal criticism.

EXTERNAL CRITICISM

External criticism evaluates a nursing theory as it relates to the real world of man, nursing, and health. In external criticism, theorists and critics generally agree that the following criteria should be achieved: reality convergence, utility, significance, and capacity for discrimination. There may be differences, however, in views concerning whether a given theory successfully achieves a given criterion. There is little consensus on two other criteria: scope and complexity. Critics take various stances on these criteria, favoring greater or lesser scope, more or less complexity.

Reality Convergence

The reality convergence is considered as it relates to principle, interpretation, and method. A theory may appear to veer significantly from the real world in one or more of these aspects.

Every theory is built on one or more essential principles. Principles are the crucial premises of a theory. As a theory develops, the conclusions of earlier arguments often become the premises in later assertions, thus creating linked chains of reasoning. Nevertheless, every argument starts somewhere, with a set of premises that is not supported by prior argument. It is these premises that determine the reality convergence of the theory as to principle. Whether the original premises are the principles of the theory or whether they set the course that later leads to other, more immediate principles, it is these premises with which the question of reality convergence deals.

A reader can choose to accept or reject the basic unsupported premises of a theory. That a set of premises appears to be self-evident to a theorist does not mean that every reader will see it that way. Take, for example, Newman's (1986) expanding consciousness. If one holds a firm opinion that consciousness does not expand, then—for that reader—Newman's theory lacks reality convergence. Because the principle of expanding consciousness underlies the rest of the theory, none of it can be accepted if this basic principle is not accepted as a real statement about the human. Thus, reality convergence has to do with whether the basic premises of a theory are accepted or rejected. Notice that this component of external criticism allows for more disagreement than is the case for most criteria of internal criticism. Although all readers would agree that the basic premises of a theory must be adequate to serve as a base for theory development (internal criticism), there is little likelihood that each reader will agree on whether any particular set of premises does or does not converge with her notion of reality.

Interpretation tells what sort of nursing world the theorist perceives. Does the theorist's perception of the nursing world conform with that of the reader's? Johnson's (1980) world of behavior as the setting for nursing is a good example. For many nurses, patient *behavior* simply does not reflect the world of nursing.

Reality may refer to what is perceived to be man, health, or nursing. One critic might judge a theory to be deficient if it takes a reductionist view of *man*—for example, explaining him on the basis of stimuli and responses—if that critic has a conflicting, holistic view of man. Similarly, another critic may fault a theory for having an illness-based concept of *health*, if that critic has a strong personal commitment to well care.

Judgments of reality convergence also include disagreements about method. For example, some nurses are uncomfortable with a theory if its method does not readily lend itself to research by the so-called scientific method. Some reject the dialectic methodology on this basis. Of course, some would argue that it is possible to subject conclusions reached by dialectic reasoning to research in problematic or logistic modes. We will address this notion in Chapter 20. In looking at the criterion of reality convergence, it is important to recognize that any given theory can be negated by viewing that theory in light of a different principle, interpretation, or method. If the critic *assumes* that a logistic approach is the only acceptable method, then she simply rejects every nonlogistic theory as failing to reflect reality. Similarly, a critic committed to a problematic method will reject a nonproblematic method. There is no higher court of appeals to which such basic disagreements can be referred.

Utility

The criterion of utility requires that a nursing theory be useful to the practitioner in her work, be it nursing practice, education, research, or administration. A nursing theory should structure the work of the practicing nurse, giving her a frame of reference from which to view patients and from which to make patient care decisions. For the nurse educator, a theory should provide the basis for curriculum organization as well as indicate appropriate methods of teaching. A theory has utility for the nurse researcher if it suggests important subject matter for investigation and appropriate methods of enquiry. And a theory has utility for the nurse administrator if it guides the organization of the nursing department and delivery of nursing care services. If a theory is too esoteric to be applied in day-to-day operations and decisions, then it fails to meet the criterion of utility.

If a theory is to be usable, its selected concepts must be pragmatic, that is, they take on meaning in the world of extant nursing activities. One might, for example, examine King's (1981) principle of transaction: an agreement reached between patient and nurse in relation to any subject matter. One might criticize this principle as lacking utility for the care of many patients (e.g., the comatose, the irrational, or the newborn).

Suppose King were to respond to this criticism with an argument that her theory was not meant to cover all nursing occasions? This would shift the argument from one of utility to one of scope.

Utility requires that the concepts of a theory be operationalized. Here, some might take issue with Rogers's (1990, p. 8) principle of *resonancy* (continuous change from lower to higher frequency wave patterns in human and environmental fields). If a nurse could not conceptualize how that principle could direct her practice, it would lack utility. Of course, another nurse might understand the principle in a way that allowed her to use it in clinical practice. The question of utility depends on who can use what and how.

To exhibit utility, a theory must direct work in extant settings. Its terms and concepts must be operationalized in ways that allow its application, and that application must facilitate the nursing activities rather than hinder them.

Significance

A theory meets the criterion of significance if it addresses essential, not peripheral, issues in nursing and contributes to the development of nursing knowledge. The criterion of significance has both these elements. The first might be coined the *so what factor*. Often one hears a theory explained, finds no fault with its internal structure, sees its applicability to practice, yet is tempted to ask, So what? Usually this happens when the selected subject matter of the theory is peripheral to one's concept of what nursing is really about. Because nursing is such a complex phenomenon, it is not surprising that some authors opt to deal with trivialized concepts that are easily explained and manipulated.

The second element contained in the criterion of significance is that of the theory's research potential, that is, its potential for expanding nursing knowledge. If a theory is significant, it lends itself to further nursing research. Ellis (1968), in a classic piece on characteristics of theories, noted,

> Another characteristic of significant theories is that they are capable of generating a great deal of new information. Hypotheses which are highly probable may be so simply because they state what is apparent empirically and contribute little that is new. A theory that generates many hypotheses, even some without high probability, or some that are difficult to test, can contribute significantly to understanding (p. 221).

Sometimes, when theories are criticized as failing to lend themselves to further research, the fault may lie in the critic's narrow view of research methods rather than in the theory itself. New perceptions on research methods have greatly enhanced researchability of many theories.

The criterion of significance, then, is met when a theory is such that the research stemming from it has potential for predicting and controlling those factors that compose the essential aspects of nursing. A significant theory addresses essential, not peripheral, phenomena.

Discrimination

Another important criterion for a nursing theory is its capacity to discriminate. Does the theory differentiate nursing from other health professions on the one hand and from other caring–tending acts on the other? A theory that discriminates bounds its subject matter definitively. Discrimination is important in a practice discipline that draws on knowledge from so many other fields. If, for example, the nurse is acting *as a nurse* and not as a pharmacologist when she administers a medication, the discriminating nursing theory will enable one to explain why. Similarly, a discriminating theory would enable one to determine if a triage nurse were acting *as a nurse* or as a substitute physician.

Obviously, no two theories will include exactly the same phenomena within the given boundaries of nursing. The important point is that the boundaries be precise and clear, so that it is possible to make judgments, placing extant acts and practices inside or outside of the prescribed boundaries.

Two further criteria are important for external criticism of a theory, although there is little consensus on them: scope and complexity. Both scope and complexity may be seen as continuums, with various theorists opting for different places on them.

Scope of Theory

Authors differ about whether a nursing theory should have a broad or limited scope (conceived of as two general locations on the continuum). At one stage, the argument tended to be either/or. Now, most nurses recognize that there is place for theory development all along the continuum. The chief quality affected by scope is the depth of the theory. One can be more detailed about a theory designed to cover a limited practice—say gerontologic nursing—than when speaking for every kind of nursing imaginable.

The narrower the theory, the more potential it has for guidance; the wider the theory, the more global its terms and meanings. Obviously, the ideal would be a theory that covered all kinds of nursing yet was highly detailed in its formulation.

The scope issue will press us eventually to consider whether nursing represents a single discipline or a combination of disciplines. Will nursing be able to develop a theory that functions optimally for such diverse nursing domains as public health, psychiatric nursing, and acute care nursing? Is it even necessary? The question of utility may interact with questions of scope. If a specific theory is more useful, should a nurse in a specialty practice use a less effective wide-scope theory on principle? It does not seem to make sense.

Complexity

The criterion of complexity for a theory may be seen as opposing another criterion—that of parsimony. The argument *for* complexity in a theory is that it allows for explanation and interrelationship of more variables. Complexity enables a theory to account for the richness of its subject matter. On the other hand, the criterion of parsimony strives to limit theory elements, to streamline. Parsimony requires that the fewest possible variables be selected as descriptive and explanatory components. It has the advantage of clearly separating figure and background, of setting the critical elements of nursing in relief so that they are more easily perceived. Parsimony and complexity can be seen as opposite poles of a continuum. Yet there are times when a complex idea can be expressed in parsimonious terms. Einstein's basic theory ($E = Mc^2$) is parsimonious in the extreme, yet it represents a complex set of ideas. The balance between complexity and parsimony must be dictated by the inherent nature of nursing as perceived by the nurse theorist.

OTHER EVALUATIVE CRITERIA

This book divides evaluative criteria into those appropriate for internal and external criticism. Other theory critics elaborate different lists of criteria and different methods for evaluating theories. The reader should explore these alternate formulations as well.

Meleis (1991), for example, adds an interesting criterion called the *circle of contagiousness* (pp. 232–233). By this, she means whether, and to what degree, a theory is adopted by others. This might be called the *factor of geographic spread*. Only time will tell whether popularity and a theory's caliber coincide, but it is certainly a criterion worth assessing.

Chinn and Kramer (1991) have a parsimonious set of criteria for evaluating theories: clarity, simplicity, generality, accessibility, and importance. Clarity, for these authors mean essentially the same thing it means in this book. Their notion of simplicity refers to the number of components and relationships in a theory, whereas generality refers to the scope of events covered by the theory. Accessibility tests the extent to which empiric indicators can be identified and projected outcomes are attainable. Importance refers to the extent to which the theory has clinical significance (pp. 128–139). Whatever schema one elects to follow, the important thing is that a theory be seriously studied rather than accepted without deliberation. The more theories that a person evaluates, the easier the task becomes.

SUMMARY

This chapter examines the ways of passing judgment on a theory and deems this a valid activity. In judging a theory, however, one needs to differentiate between aspects of personal preference and elements of flawed thinking on the part of a theorist. Separating internal from external criticism assists in this endeavor. In addition, the separation encourages more vigorous thinking on the part of the evaluator.

This chapter gives the reader criteria for both internal and external analysis. The reader should appreciate that performance on one criterion may affect judgments made about others. For example, if the clarity of a theory is poor, it may be impossible to evaluate other criteria with precision.

The reader will need to recognize personal preferences that bias her evaluation of a theory. For example, a reader who detests the New Age movement may have difficulty suspending that judgment in reading a New Age theory. Not only can a reader have preferences concerning a theory, but she may have preferences concerning evaluative criteria. For example, different degrees of parsimony and complexity appeal to different people.

None of this is to say that theories should not be judged. Indeed, if nursing has erred, it has been in the failure to criticize. Criticism need not be seen in a negative light. A concise evaluation of the present formulation may be the first step in improving a theory.

REFERENCES

Chinn, P. L., & Kramer, M. K. (1991). *Theory and nursing: A systematic approach* (3rd ed.). St. Louis, MO: Mosby Year Book.

Copi, I. M. (1982). *Introduction to logic* (6th ed.). New York: Macmillan.

Ellis, R. (1968). Characteristics of significant theories. *Nursing Research, 3*, 217–222.

Johnson, D. E. (1980). The behavioral system model for nursing. In J. P. Riehl & C. Roy (Eds.), *Conceptual models for nursing practice* (2nd ed., pp. 207–216). New York: Appleton-Century-Crofts.

King, I. M. (1981). *A theory for nursing: Systems, concepts, process.* New York: Wiley.

Meleis, A. I. (1991). *Theoretical nursing: Development and progress* (2nd ed.). Philadelphia: J. B. Lippincott.

Newman, M. A. (1986). *Health as expanding consciousness.* St. Louis, MO: C. V. Mosby.

Rogers, M. E. (1990). Nursing: Science of unitary, irreducible, human beings: Update 1990. In E.A.M. Barrett (Ed.) *Visions of Rogers' science-based nursing* (pp. 5–11). New York: National League for Nursing.

Rubin, R. (1968). A theory of clinical nursing. *Nursing Research, 3*, 210–212.

14 Focus on Environment

Although every nursing theory of necessity gives some consideration to the patient's environment, there are several in which environment is the central focus. Nurses often trace their interest in environment back to Florence Nightingale. Indeed, she must have been as much sanitary engineer as nurse. Much of the text in her *Notes on Nursing* (reissued in 1992) is devoted to improvements in the patient's environment. For example, she spoke of the "health of houses," identifying five essential points: (1) pure air, (2) pure water, (3) efficient drainage, (4) cleanliness, and (5) light (p. 14).

As Schuyler (1992) summarized in that reissue,

> Nightingale's concern for the health of others was not restricted to the Army. In the ten years after the Crimean War, she worked to reform civilian hospitals and workhouse infirmaries in England; to improve health and sanitation in India and other British colonies; and to establish the first professional schools for nurses and midwives (p. 8).

Environmental reform was the crux of most of these diverse activities. Of course, the meaning of *environment* changes with each nurse theorist, but nurses have sustained that interest in environment. The environments range from a community health perspective, to a notion of mind as environment, to a perception of culture as the important environmental factor, to an even more global concept of environment.

In the United States, public health nursing has always been associated with the environment. Indeed, the early public health nurses dealt with environmental concerns not unlike those faced by Nightingale herself: unsanitary conditions, nutritional failures, industrial hazards, and ill health due to both poverty and ignorance.

Today, we have two environmental models that follow in this tradition: the public health nursing model and the community health

Barbara J. Stevens Barnum: NURSING THEORY: ANALYSIS, APPLICATION, EVALUATION, FOURTH EDITION. © 1994, 1990, 1984, 1979 J.B. Lippincott.

nursing model. Rothman (1990) has differentiated between them this way:

> Community health nursing practice concentrates on the direct care of individuals, families, and groups; the community is a client to the degree that it impacts on the direct care of individuals, families, and groups. Public health nursing is directed toward legal mandates to protect health and programs for specific segments of the population. . . .
>
> The public health nurse employs a method/process directed toward identification of high-risk groups and collaborates with multidisciplinary teams in planning and coordinating programs and services to address actual and potential health problems (p. 418).

Rothman differentiated nursing of people in communities from the nursing of substandard communities themselves. This to not say that everyone agrees with Rothman's differentiations, nor do programs in public health always opt for one model to the exclusion of the other. In many educational programs—and community health nursing positions as well—one finds combined models.

By whatever name, public health/community health nursing is one model of care that looks beyond the patient's immediate environment (often perceived as hospital, home, long-term care facility); that is, it sees environment as more than the place where the patient is physically housed.

We will look at two other environmentally driven types of theory in this chapter: transcultural theory and feminist theory. These two forms share a conviction that the theories focused only on a patient's immediate environment miss the point. Both direct their followers to look beyond the sick room and both judge the focus of public health nursing to be too narrow. Beyond that agreement, they diverge radically.

TRANSCULTURAL NURSING

Leininger (1991) is credited with making transcultural nursing a major theme in nursing theory. With her anthropologic background, it is not surprising that she found nursing care to suffer when the nurse failed to appreciate the patient's culture and the meanings that culture attributes to illnesses and treatment.

For Leininger, the cultural dimension is imposed on a strong commitment to a care philosophy. Welding the two concepts together, she has made nurses aware of the importance of considering a patient's culture in trying to help him. In essence, Leininger has encouraged two trends in nursing: first, a concentrated study of selected cultures by nurses intending to work with those populations, and second, the development among nurses of a general sensitivity to the fact that all people have cultural patterns and meanings that should be considered in developing plans of care.

Leininger's theory was briefly reviewed in Chapter 6, and the reader may wish to refresh her memory of it before reading further. Many of Leininger's (1991) assumptive premises deal with the cultural aspect of nursing, including the following:

- Every human culture has generic (lay, folk, or indigenous) care knowledge and practices and usually professional care knowledge and practices that vary transculturally.
- Clients who experience nursing care that fails to be reasonably congruent with the client's beliefs, values, and caring lifeways will show signs of cultural conflicts, noncompliance, stresses, and ethical or moral concerns (p. 45).

Additionally, in her transcultural research, Leininger (1991) found the following:

- There are more signs of diversities than universalities among the 54 cultures, and especially between Western and non–Western cultures.
- Culture care meanings and practices are difficult to tease out largely because they are embedded in the social structure, in non–Western cultures especially in kinship, religious beliefs, and political factors; whereas in Western cultures care is viewed largely as high-tech tasks, cost factors, political decisions, and problems with language to understand clients' care needs (p. 57).

Nurses educated in Leininger's and other transcultural programs have been sensitized to the needs of patients from other cultures. In a world that grows constantly smaller and more mobile, the message is timely. For these nurses, the patient's environment, namely, his culture, *is* the message, and when a nurse cannot read the message, care efforts may fail.

FEMINIST THEORY IN NURSING

Although one might assume that Leininger's position could hardly be sullied, that is not the case. Many feminists insist that her approach to environment is passive. Leininger, in effect, says: Get to know the patient's culture, honor its precepts, its lifeways.

Feminist theories also focus on a notion of environment, but they take a highly active stance. The feminist perspective starts with a notion that things are wrong and they need changing. Many, but not all, of the things wrong have to do with mistreatment of women. Feminist theories range from putting the spotlight on a single nation to a viewpoint considering all the nations of the earth as environment.

Unlike Leininger, they see the selected environment as a first concern and more important than the one-to-one care arena, not simply as a vehicle for making one-to-one care more effective. In effect, the nation or its government may be the patient. Obviously, the two concerns are not mutually exclusive, but most feminists have a strong commitment to placing the macroscopic vision before and above the one-to-one perspective.

In essence, they have a trickle-down philosophy: change the big things first, then the smaller ones will follow. Watson is one of the few feminists who wrote with equal facility in both camps, that is, the feminist perspective (1990) and the one-to-one care ideology (1988).

Feminists often criticize theories such as Watson's care theory for failing to have what they see as the larger vision (the world, instead of the individual). Watson could give a good argument against that criticism, because she sees the world and human beings in a different context—at least when she is writing care theory. Chinn (1989) also has managed at times to balance the microcosms and macrocosms.

FEMINIST POLITICS

Over its long history, nursing's association with feminism has been challenging, to say the least. One would imagine that a profession so heavily dominated by women would be ripe for feminist concerns. Yet in some ways nursing has been a conservative profession—having been long dominated by a male-controlled health care industry as Ashley (1977) maintained in her classic book on the subject. Furthermore, the nonnursing feminist press and major feminist organizations have often taken positions condemning nursing for its conservatism, or worse, suggesting that ambitious women would select medicine over nursing as a career goal.

Some feminists perceive an inherent conflict between the values of feminism and the values expressed in caring. Condon (1992) explained the feminist concern that any feminine role perceived as following a caring model puts the carers at risk of exploitation by those for whom they care, thereby reinforcing the oppressive expectation that women should be selfless carers (p. 17).

Nevertheless, the voice of feminism is alive and well in nursing, with nurses voicing positions ranging from modest to radical. Moccia

(1990), one of the advocates for a strong feminist base for nursing, has challenged the profession in this manner:

> If nurses are to become active participants in bringing society to a new reality, if we are to fulfill the role of transformative intellectuals, then we will have to redefine ourselves and our institutions. As we find ways to break the tentacles of the patriarchy and to erode its base, we will obviously find ourselves in new relationships (p. 75).

Often the feminist position has a sense of rage underlying its positions and theories. Moccia (1990), again, illustrated this point:

> There is too much that is unconscionable and cries out for relief—so much that we are left shaking and trembling and close to being paralyzed by moral outrage. The dark motif of the patriarchy encourages a sense of futility, desperation, and of irreparable ruptures between private lives and public actions (p. 76).

All feminist philosophies espouse the importance of gender equity and all try to raise the social consciousness of women and men in recognizing sexist inequities in the society. The inequities addressed are as variable as are the countries in which feminists speak, write, and become politically active. The use of sexist language has always been one of the tamer themes, and Sampsell (1990) discussed the subject in typical feminist fashion:

> The patriarchal view of woman as a subspecies of man shows readily in the contemporary experience. Common language is rife with examples such as the generic use of man and masculine pronouns to represent all human beings (e.g., the paradigm that depicts nursing expertise in the areas of Man, Health and Environment); the lack of gender fairness (e.g., man and woman are parallel terms, whereas man and wife defines the man as an individual and the woman only in relationship to him) and the negative connotation reserved for words that depict feminine traits. . . (p. 244).

Although creating a sensitivity to language is on most feminist agendas, political action to right societal insults against women is a higher priority.

ECOFEMINISM

The newest version of feminism is one that combines the feminist perspective with an ecologic viewpoint (ecofeminism). From an ecofeminist perspective, what is cared for, cared about, is the planet, the earth itself, including its populations. The proposed solutions advocate advancing feminist power and preserving ecology at the same time. Obviously the ecologic and the feminist viewpoints can be and, in many cases, are separated. However, at present, we see a strong tendency to combine the two factions.

In most versions, the ecofeminist viewpoint is not set in the so-called New Age world paradigm; instead, its ideology represents a counterculture position against the social and political factions in power in various governments worldwide. Although their position is coined against the acts of these ruling powers, the view of the world (context in our terms) is similar. Those in power and the feminists see the same world; they simply interpret it differently and would like it to be managed in different ways.

Kleffel (1991) described the ecofeminist position as one that sees the fate of the human species and the planet at stake. She further postulated that no male-led revolution will counteract the present horrors of overpopulation and destruction of natural resources (p. 7). This linked concern for the natural world and for the abuses of a male-run society is typical of the ecofeminist position.

Some nurses are uncomfortable with the tactics of assertive feminists. True, some feminists can be strident, taking positions that seem harsh. These feminists would claim that their tactics are shaped by today's world and that they have little choice if they are to make an impact. Feminist choices involve not only matters of tactics but selections of themes as well. As has ever been the case, it is not always possible to serve a larger cause and the individual simultaneously. And where choice must be made, most nurses in the feminist camp opt for the macrocosmic view over the one-to-one-ideology.

Nurse ecofeminists (or simply feminists, for that matter) decry that the typical nursing theory takes a one-nurse-to-one-patient perspective. They object to the environment's being conceived as the patient's immediate surroundings. Both of these positions, they assert, narrow one's perspective and keep nursing from addressing its true subject matter: the larger social, political, and ecologic global picture. The feminist perspective makes political reform the immediate, not a tangential aim of nursing. This represents a radical change in content from other theories we have examined.

FEMINISTS: NOT ALL ALIKE

Kleffel (1991) differentiated four types of contemporary feminism: (1) liberal feminism, (2) radical feminism, (3) traditional Marxist feminism, and (4) socialist feminism (p. 7). Her list should serve to remind us that feminists, even among nurses, are not all of a kind. It is true, however, that some of the feminists once classified as

Marxist or socialist have shifted their interest to the ecologic, not surprising in a world in which so many communist and socialist states have recently fallen, bringing the political form into question.

The linking of a feminist agenda to an ecologic agenda, for the most part, simply broadens feminist goals. The earlier focus on gender equity has not been sacrificed. Indeed, the growing sensitivity to harassment in the workplace has increased the zeal of this pursuit by most feminists. Battling violence against women remains a major effort on the feminist agenda. Another issue of major importance—the lack of attention given to women's diseases or women's fate when contracting any disease—has received an important boost by new requirements that federally sponsored research include women as study subjects.

Whatever the focus—ecology, women's rights, women's health, or societal failures—feminists of all persuasions tend to focus on political action. They recognize that government is the major decision maker on these issues. For feminist nurses, the appropriate subject matter (content) for nursing is politics. Achieving the desired political world is seen as a prerequisite for the hands-on care that is the first concern in most nursing theories.

The failure of feminists to focus first and foremost on the quality of one-to-one care is confusing to some nurses who have internalized that role as their chief function. In essence, although most nurses support feminist goals, many would assert that the feminist political focus, worthy though it may be, simply is not nursing. Other nurses are bothered that some feminist groups favor political revolution to reform, but feminist groups are far from agreement on their political goals and tactics.

Many people think of feminist theories as holistic, but that is not always the case. The confusion is probably because their common subject matter (the state of the country or world) seems large. But the approach, at least in the nursing literature, is seldom holistic. Instead, feminists seem interested in analyzing the parts (political decisions); analyzing the infrastructures of a society; and intervening in them—in essence, a view in which the whole is known through its parts.

In contrast, Marxist feminists, when they are consistent to original Marxian principles, may be following a dialectic thought pattern in which the world is seen as evolving, moving through an inevitable series of thesis, antithesis, and synthesis. Moccia is a good example of a feminist who is sensitive to the dialectic thought process. Many others, however, have assumed the feminist causes without adopting the Hegelian/Marxist dialectic.

SUMMARY

There are many nursing theories that concentrate on environment, starting with Nightingale, leading forward into our own time. Some of the theories look at environment as it relates directly to the patient; some view the environment itself as the patient, that is, as the focus for their attention.

Many environmental theories (from Nightingale to the feminists) could be characterized as crusader theories. Simply, they aim to change things, whether the environment that is pursued is ecologic, social, or political. Yet other theories (like Leininger's) are more passive—not that she hesitated in setting out to change major environmental hazards. But on the whole, Leininger and the transcultural nursing movement see environment more as a tool to be used in providing better one-to-one care.

The present era is ripe for the development of more environmental theories of nursing, particularly as care becomes distributed, that is, offered in many settings other than the acute care hospital. Although there is no single environmental nursing theory that can give the forerunners (that is, nursing process/diagnosis/intervention and holistic theories) a run for their money, the creation of a compelling theory in this area would be a welcome addition.

REFERENCES

Ashley, J. A. (1977). *Hospitals, paternalism, and the role of the nurse.* New York: Teachers College Press.

Chinn, P. L. (1989). Nursing patterns of knowing and feminist thought. *Nursing & Health Care, 2,* 71–75.

Condon, E. H. (1992). Nursing and the caring metaphor: Gender and political influences on an ethics of care. *Nursing Outlook, 1,* 14–19.

Kleffel, D. (1991). An ecofeminist analysis of nursing knowledge. *Nursing Forum, 4,* 5–18.

Leininger, M. M. (1991). The theory of culture care diversity and universality. In M. M. Leininger (Ed.), *Culture care diversity & universality: A theory of nursing* (pp. 5–68). New York: National League for Nursing.

Moccia, P. (1990). Re-claiming our communities. *Nursing Outlook, 2,* 73–76.

Nightingale, F. (1992). *Notes on nursing* (reissue). Philadelphia: J. B. Lippincott.

Rothman, N. L. (1990). Toward description: Public health nursing and community health nursing are different. *Nursing & Health Care, 9,* 481–483.

Sampsell, C. M. (1990). The influence of feminist philosophy on nursing practice. *Image, 4,* 243–247.

Schuyler, C. B. (1992). Florence Nightingale. In F. Nightingale (Ed.) with D. P. Carroll, *Notes on nursing* (reissue, pp. 4–17). Philadelphia: J. B. Lippincott.

Watson, J. (1988). *Nursing: Human science and human care: A theory of nursing.* New York: National League for Nursing.

Watson, J. (1990). The moral failure of the patriarchy. *Nursing Outlook, 2,* 62–66.

BIBLIOGRAPHY

Anderson, J. M. (1991). Reflexivity in fieldwork: Toward a feminist epistemology. *Image, 2,* 115–118.

Bullough, V. (1990). Nightingale, nursing and harassment. *Image, 1,* 4–7.

Chinn, P. L., & Wheeler, C. E. (1985), Feminism and nursing: Can nursing afford to remain aloof from the women's movement? *Nursing Outlook, 2,* 74–77.

Forman, F. J., & Sowton, C. (Eds.). (1989). *Taking our time: Feminist perspectives on temporality.* New York: Pergamon.

Gilligan, C. (1982). *In a different voice: Psychological theory and women's development.* Cambridge, MA: Harvard University Press.

Kleffel, D. (1991). Rethinking the environment as a domain of nursing knowledge. *Advances in Nursing Science, 1,* 40–51.

Leininger, M. M. (Ed.). (1988). *Care: Discovery and uses in clinical and community nursing.* Detroit, MI: Wayne State University Press.

Mason, D. J., Backer, B. A., & Georges, C. A. (1991). Toward a feminist model for the political empowerment of nurses. *Image, 2,* 72–77.

Moccia, P. (1988). At the faultline: Social activism and caring. *Nursing Outlook, 1,* 30–33.

Moccia, P. (1991). Nursing education as social reform. *Dean's Notes, 1,* 1–3.

Polusny, S. M. (1989). Feminist friendship: Isabel Hampton Robb, Lavinia Lloyd Dock and Mary Adelaide Nutting. *Image, 2,* 64–68.

Reverby, S. M. (1987). *Ordered to care: The dilemma of American nursing, 1850–1945.* New York: Cambridge University Press.

Vicinus, M., & Nergaard, B. (1989). *Ever yours, Florence Nightingale: Selected letters.* Cambridge, MA: Harvard University Press.

15 *Common Themes in Nursing Theory*

This chapter summarizes and examines the common themes in nursing theory—not in an attempt to synthesize them, but to identify the different subject matters and approaches. We will produce a map of topics and viewpoints, not a theory of nursing.

The questions to be asked are: What can be gained by taking this subject matter or this approach for nursing theory? Which topics and which approaches are compatible and which contradictory if used within a single theory formulation?

SUBJECT MATTER OF NURSING THEORY

Most theories take as their primary subject matter man, the nurse, environment, health, or their interfaces. Variations on these themes include the nursing act, man–environment, man in groups, man in organizations, man as he participates in God, and the health care system—to name only a few. Each of these subject matters, as we have already seen, can be perceived in an infinite number of ways.

Man-Centered Theories of Nursing

An underlying assumption in man-centered theories of nursing is that to know man is to be able to infer what nursing is required. A major question for theories with this theme is whether nursing's subject matter is the *total* man or some *component* of his being. Furthermore, if nursing is applied to the total man, one must ask if that means man as an indivisible whole or if it means all the units composing his totality (e.g., psyche and soma; psychological, physio-

Barbara J. Stevens Barnum: NURSING THEORY:
ANALYSIS, APPLICATION, EVALUATION, FOURTH EDITION.
© 1994, 1990, 1984, 1979 J.B. Lippincott.

logic, and spiritual components; the various body systems taken together; man's structure and function; or some other variation on man's components). If, on the other hand, nursing is responsible for only some (but not all) components, which components fall inside of nursing's domain?

Man-centered theories also should declare *when* the total or partial man requires nursing. In some theories, man is labeled a patient when a health deficiency occurs. Other theories expand the category to include persons vulnerable to health deficits not yet manifest. Some theories consider every living person as patient for a lifetime.

In many New Age theories, for example, nursing is an act of assisting in human development (expanding consciousness, extending self-mastery). These theories imply that nursing is an ongoing activity that man needs at every phase of life, regardless of his particular health status. When nursing is seen as always applicable, it tends to be equated with meeting all human needs. In other cases, it is tightly tied to developmental needs, with "needs" being interpreted from traditional patterns, like Erikson (1963), to transpersonal patterns, like Wilber (1980).

Notice the boundary issues that arise here if nurses fail to differentiate themselves from others who also might see themselves as guardians of development, such as psychiatrists, developmental psychologists, transpersonal psychologists, or clergymen.

When the need for nursing is perceived as intermittent, it is usually limited to the meeting of health-related needs. A theory should identify the phenomena that initiate the need for nursing (e.g., stress or strain, disequilibrium or ineffective adaptation, a deficit, incapacity, dysfunctional or deviant behavior, disharmony, disease, and the like).

Sometimes it is not the individual man who is the subject matter of a theory. There are numerous *plural man* theories in which a theorist claims that her patient is a group or community of men. When only one of these alternatives is singled out, the theorist is usually on firm ground. But when man, man in groups, *and* man in larger communities are all asserted to be legitimate subjects of the same theory, look skeptically on the claim.

Often this is a slogan that, once said, is ignored. Watch to see if the theorist ever uses the larger sense of patient in her examples and explanations. Suppose, for example, that her patient is defined by his disequilibrium. Does she ever tell how to recognize disequilibrium in a group or community? Are her examples of care applicable to the larger sense of patient or only to the one-on-one situation? It is not wrong to have a subject matter of plural man, but it *is* wrong if it is not carried through in the resultant theory.

Man–Other Units as Theory Subject Matter

In man–other units, man is still the subject matter, but he is seen through his blending with and participation in something else. (Some would consider that the plural man theories just discussed fit into this category.) The "other" that is combined with man may be any sort of social, political, geographic, or conceptual entity.

Man in relation to family is one such unit. Notice there are two ways to consider man and his family. Man-as-a-family-member (husband, father, mother, child) would compose a man–other unit. In other cases, the entire family unit becomes the patient (rather than any member of it being singled out). The psychiatric nurse therapist, for example, might take the family as a whole as her unit of analysis and therapy. For a comparative view of different approaches to family therapy, see Whall (1980).

The same difference applies to notions of public health or community health nursing. Man-in-the-community is a man–other unit, whereas the community as patient could qualify as an environmental theory instead.

Sometimes the conjoined unit is much larger than the man–family or man–community unit. Man–environment or even man–universe theories are popular. The new paradigm theories specialize in these "larger than life" perspectives. Some religious theories take a similar perspective, for example, Longway's (1970) focus on the man–God interface could be conceived to qualify here. In man–other theories, nursing may prescribe intervention in either man, the "other," or both.

The Nurse as Subject Matter

Some theories take the nurse rather than man (the patient) as the focal subject matter. The approach varies widely, from looking at roles performed, to identifying tasks, to examining the motivation of the nurse. It is not uncommon for theorists who use an operational methodology to view nursing in terms of role, and it is not uncommon for caring theories to view the nurse through her motivation. The nursing process identifies the nurse through what she does, that is, her activities, both intellectual and psychomotor. When nonnurses study nursing, they frequently equate nursing with merely the psychomotor tasks that are self-evident and open to observation.

Sometimes the nurse is defined by her credentials or licenses—as a registered professional nurse, as a baccalaureate-prepared nurse, or as a certified midwife, for example. This is a legalistic answer to the problem of definition. Other times, nurse is perceived to include all members of the nursing staff (aides, licensed practical nurses). In some theories, the term *nurse* may be applied to anyone who completes acts of a specified nature, with or without educational or experiential qualifications.

Considering Patient and Nurse Together

It is common, though not essential, that the patient and the nurse act out of reciprocal, complementary principles. For example, Johnson's (1980) patient is motivated by a disturbance in one or more behavioral system, perhaps a frustrated drive. Her nurse, reciprocally, is an external regulatory force who aims to restore or attain behavioral system balance and stability.

In Levine's (1971) theory, the patient *adapts*, whereas the nurse *conserves* (she conserves those patient adaptations that are seen as productive). In Hall's (1966) theory, the nurse *mirrors* (reflects back the patient's own feelings), whereas the patient *masters* (his feelings, his self-control).

In Roy's (1980) theory, the patient *responds to stimuli*, whereas the nurse *manipulates stimuli*. Even Orlando's (1990) theory has reciprocal principles, if a bit more complicated than many of previously discussed theories. The nurse observes the patient's behavior, interprets it, then checks her reaction with the patient. Only after the patient confirms or clarifies the meaning of the behavior, does she act on the behavior to solve the patient's problem. We could summarize the system as patient action, nurse reaction, nurse–patient validation, and nurse action.

In a few theories, the patient and the nurse operate based on the same principle rather than complementary principles. In Orem's (1985) theory, for example, both act out of self-care agency. The nurse's justification for taking over the patient's self-care is the patient's incapacity to do so. The principle from which they act, however, remains the same: self-care.

A few theories focus so exclusively on one polarity of the relationship (either the patient or the nurse) that they say little about the other aspect. One might, for example, consider Rogers's work as one that focuses primarily on the patient, that is, the nature of what it is to be a human (unitary man). Rogers's (1990) principles (resonancy, helicy, integrality) rest in unitary man, not in the nurse-as-nurse nor in the nursing act (as discrete from other human actions).

In contrast, Benner's (1984) theory focuses on the nurse, not the patient, identifying the following seven domains of nursing practice: (1) the helping role, (2) the teaching–coaching function, (3) the diagnostic and patient-monitoring function, (4) effective management of rapidly changing situations, (5) the administration and monitoring of therapeutic interventions and regimens, (6) the monitoring of and assurance of the quality of health care practices, and (7) organizational and work-role competencies (pp. 44–46). Although these actions rest in the nurse, they are not principles as was the case in the examples cited earlier. Someday, someone may mine Benner's material for the principles of nursing action expressed through these domains.

For most theories, it is possible to represent the nurse–patient relationship as a sequential triad: (1) the patient's undesirable, initial status; (2) the nursing act; and (3) the patient's desirable status (goal or end point). Some examples follow:

Hall
1. decreased self-control
2. mirroring-nurturing
3. self-mastery

Levine
1. disequilibrium
2. conservation
3. equilibrium

Roy
1. responses exceeding the adaptation level
2. manipulation of stimuli
3. responses within the adaptation level

Orem
1. (decreased) self-care
2. (substituted) self-care
3. (resumed) self-care

Notice that these triads shift from patient to nurse to patient. When the patient also assists in effecting his cure or care, such as with Levine's patient, one could build another triad exclusive to the patient. For Levine's patient, that would be (1) disequilibrium, (2) adaptation, and (3) equilibrium.

IN THE NEW PARADIGM

The newer developmental theories often do not show such a shift in principle from patient to nurse. Instead, as Watson (1988) has said, "The agent of change in this work is viewed as the individual patient, but the nurse can be a coparticipant in change through the human care process." (p. 74) Or as Quinn (1992) has claimed, the nurse is the midwife to healing (p. 28); she is an environment for the patient, a space where there the resonance of two people interacts during healing (p. 34).

Theories in the new paradigm usually see the patient as the main agent, the nurse as helper. A few New Age theories would be classified as patient focused, but the newer ones usually focus on the interaction (like Quinn and Watson). Yet even with a focus on the interaction, the patient is weightier than the nurse. The nurse helps build the interaction, but the patient remains captain of the relationship. Quinn's midwife example works well in describing the power relations of the situation.

In analyzing and understanding any nursing theory, it is important to understand where the focus lies. Is the author interested in telling nurses what to do? Is the author interested in understanding the patient? Obviously, these are not incompatible goals, but it is typical for one aspect to be stressed, the other not.

When the patient is the focus, the theorist might argue that adequate knowledge of the patient makes the necessary nursing care self-evident. Whether this is true depends on the author's conceptualization of the patient. In a physiologically based conceptualization of the patient, the thesis might hold. On the whole, patient-based theories have a certain humanitarian appeal because they start and end with the patient foremost in mind.

Theories that rest heavily on the nursing side of the equation often have actional principles. They have intrinsic appeal to the young nurse learner for the simple reason that they give strong directives, that is, they tell her what to do. Although most theories of this sort deal with the nurse's overt actions, others focus instead on her thought processes.

Theories in the new paradigm show an interesting development in relation to the patient–nurse duality. Originally, most focused heavily on the nature of man—like Rogers's (1970) original work. Now the theories are developing in two directions, some focusing on the nature of the interrelationship between patient and nurse, others developing sets of nursing interventions (Dossey, Keegan, Kolkmeier, & Guzzetta, 1989; Quinn, 1992). In what appears to be a more rapid pace, the Dossey and colleagues and Quinn theories are following the same pattern of development as nursing process (which preceded the work on its interventions).

NURSE–PATIENT INTERACTION AS SUBJECT MATTER

One important aspect of the nurse–patient linkage deals with interpretation. Although it is legitimate for the nurse to act on principles different from those of the patient, it is not legitimate for her to be a creature from a different world. It is poor form when a theory forgets this. Take, for example, a case in which the patient is explained entirely in terms of stimulus–response. That is certainly one valid view of man—but not if the nurse is seen as operating outside of a stimulus–response theory herself. Suppose, for example, the same author has the nurse operating in a freewill context, one in which, unlike the patient, her choices are not based on prior conditioning. Errors such as this one are easier to catch if the reader carefully considers patient and nurse together. Remember, the critical questions are: Who is the nurse? What is the nursing act? Who or what is the patient? In what way do the two interface? Which of them, if either, is the dominant theme in the given theory?

Interaction theories take as their subject matter the conceptual product of the man–nurse exchange. For example, in King's (1981) theory, the ultimate principle of *transaction* arises between patient and nurse in the midst of their agreements. In Watson's (1988) theory, a transcendent coming together is possible. In both of these illustrations, the principle attaches to the interaction, not to the patient or the nurse.

Leininger's (1991) latest theory is an interesting variation on the interaction theme. Like Roy's (1980) theory, Leininger's rests heavily on the nurse's autonomous decision making (she preserves/maintains, accommodates/negotiates, repatterns/restructures; pp. 41–42). Yet there is a requisite interaction of an unusual sort. It is not between nurse and patient but between two competing health care systems: the care of the folkways and the care of the professional caregivers. For Leininger's system to work, the professionals must resolve differences between their system and the lay system—sort of a negotiation, with the professionals negotiating from strength (their knowledge of both systems).

Because Chapter 16 deals exclusively with theories in which the principle arises *between* the patient and nurse, we will not discuss them at length in this chapter. Keep in mind, however, that the interaction is yet a third type of subject matter for nursing theory.

ENVIRONMENT AS SUBJECT MATTER

There are times when environment is taken as the primary subject matter of nursing theory. How the environment is seen can be radically different from one theory to another. It could be a community, a given social class, a health care system, a political system, or the whole earth for that matter.

As indicated in Chapter 14, in some community health approaches, a neighborhood becomes the patient, that is, the direct target of the nursing actions. In feminist theories, the political structure might be the subject matter; in ecofeminism, the planet. In essence, the environment means different things for different authors.

Most nursing theories consider environment as a subtopic, rather than the primary subject matter. Yet we have just identified two exceptions: some feminist theory and some public health conceptualizations. In both, the larger unit rather than the hands-on care unit were selected as the crux of the matter. It is assumed that resolving the macrolevel problems (however envisioned) will deter the ongoing need for one-to-one care.

Nursing administration theories also may take the health care organization as primary subject matter. However, such theories are hardly meant to replace caregiving models.

HEALTH AS THEORY SUBJECT MATTER

It is rare for *health* itself to be the primary subject of a nursing theory. Usually it is a goal, and what gets attention are the perceived ways and means. Nevertheless, it is useful to look at health as a subject matter of theory—keeping in mind that it is unlikely to be the main subject matter.

A comprehensive theory of health may include all aspects of health on an illness-to-wellness continuum. Some theories focus only on the ill-health end of that continuum. These, like Orem's (1985) theory, justify the need for a nurse by a patient's deficit.

One common tactic is to view health as some sort of equilibrium (e.g., homeostasis or homeokinesis). In models of this sort, adaptation (whatever is done to restore equilibrium) may be perceived as the function of the patient, the nurse, or both. What is kept in equilibrium may vary from physiologic, to psychological, to sociologic, to spiritual. Johnson's (1980) theory is an equilibrium model in which the subject matter (behavioral equilibrium) is unique.

One form of the equilibrium–disequilibrium theory is the theory that takes stress as its major theme. Usually theories of this sort differentiate the stressor (source) from the strain (the result in the patient). Vocabulary differs widely, however, in respect to what terms indicate these two factors. Some poorly developed theories fail to differentiate stressor and strain. See Scott, Oberst, and Dropkin (1980) for a good example of a stress theory.

Newer paradigms are more likely to see health as a state of continuous human evolution to higher and higher levels, however defined. Newman (1986) and Fitzpatrick (1983) seem more goal driven than some (toward faster rhythms or more expanded consciousness respectively). Yet even Watson (1988), who apparently progresses at a less frenetic pace, has said that "the person has one basic striving: to actualize the real self, thereby developing the spiritual essence of the self, and in the highest sense, to become more Godlike." (p. 57)

RECAPPING

One way to look at themes in nursing theory is to examine the subject matters selected by theorists. We have identified six subject matters:

1. man (as patient)
2. man as a component of some larger, more encompassing unit
3. the nurse or nursing act
4. nurse–patient interactions
5. environment
6. health

Although not all inclusive, these subject matters dominate in the majority of nursing theories. The patient, the nurse, the environment, and health (however these entities are defined) are commonplaces used in most descriptions of nursing theory. This chapter has demonstrated the diversity represented by all of these ideas. When one hears the common plea that all nursing theories are alike because they address these same subject matters, the reader will understand how deceiving that notion can be.

Approaches to the Nursing Domain

In addition to looking at what constitutes the nursing subject matter, it is important to characterize the theorist's perception of that domain. Although many classification schemes are possible, the author finds it useful to classify nursing theories according to the character of the nursing act in relation to the patient. This classification allows for the following organization of nursing theories: (1) intervention, (2) conservation, (3) substitution, (4) sustenance, and (5) enhancement.

In an *intervention theory*, the nurse actively selects variables (in the patient or in the environment) for manipulation to bring about a determined change in the present state. The change to be desired is determined by the nurse, typically using her knowledge of health, societal norms, or both. Roy (1980) and Johnson (1980) exemplify this approach.

In intervention theories, action and decision making rest heavily on the nurse as a professional. The patient tends to be treated as the object of nursing rather than as a participant in the determination of his care. References to patient participation, when they occur in such theories, tend to be slogans rather than intrinsic to theory development. Ultimately, the nurse determines and executes the proper manipulation to bring about the desired change. Intervention theories rely on the concept of professional expertise exercised by the nurse.

A *conservation theory*, in contrast, aims to preserve those beneficial aspects of the patient's present situation, especially those beneficial aspects threatened by illness, problems, or (in the case of preventive care) potential problems. Levine's (1971) early model is a good example of a conservation theory. Some public health theories rest on a conservation theory of nursing. In an era of growing public awareness of a person's responsibility for his own health, a conservation theory may provide a good fit with the social environment.

In contrast to the conservation theory, a *substitution theory* does not act by preserving what still exists, but by substituting for those capabilities the patient is no longer able to execute or no longer possesses. Here, agency resides with the patient, and nursing is a substitute for the patient's own will or intent. Agency moves from patient to nurse during the patient's incapacity.

Most substitution theories stress that the substitution be controlled, that the patient exercise his will and physical control to the greatest possible or logical extent. Undesired substitution is not inflicted on him. Nursing supplied in the absence of communication of patient intent is perceived as being what the patient would desire were he able to communicate that desire. In most substitution theories, the nurse is the patient's agent; she does not superimpose her own values, goals, and judgments for his when he is able to express them. Orem (1985) is a good example of an author who advocates a substitution theory.

Intervention and substitution theories reveal the polarities of the nurse–patient agency question, with intervention resting on the nursing agency of the professional, substitution resting on patient agency. The conservation theory, to a degree, bridges this polarity: agency rests with the nurse, but she conserves what already is inherent in the patient.

The *sustenance theory* is less concerned with impacting on the course of an illness *per se*. Instead, it focuses on enabling the patient to better endure the passage of the health insult. Focus is on support and building coping mechanisms (both psychological and physiologic).

Rubin (1968) exemplifies an author who uses a sustenance theory. She sees the goal of nursing as ego maintenance in a stressful dependency situation (p. 210). The nursing care required is determined by the degree to which the patient can or cannot cope (unassisted) with a situation at any given time.

An *enhancement theory* of nursing is one that sees nursing as a means of improving the quality of the patient's existence, either in total, in relation to health, or in relation to some specified aspect of his being. Hall (1966) and Rogers (1970) exemplified early enhancement theories, Watson (1988) and Newman (1986), later ones. Most enhancement theories are dialectic, developmental, existential, or some combination of these elements. Enhancement theories share the perception that nursing enables the patient to emerge from the health insult (in some way) stronger, better, or improved because of having experienced or overcome the health insult.

Like the intervention theory, the enhancement theory aims to produce a change for the better. Unlike the intervention theory, the nature of that enhancement remains internal to the patient rather than being specifically determined and characterized in advance by the nurse.

SUMMARY

In this chapter, we have identified common topics of and approaches to nursing theory. The perspective has not been all encompassing. But even these limited commonplaces (the various subject matters and approaches) indicate the width of perspectives and diversity of topics one finds in nursing. Taken together, these topics represent the dominant approaches to the study of nursing theory today. The area most likely to expand—seen in trends like ecofeminism—is environment as subject matter.

REFERENCES

Benner. P. (1984). *From novice to expert: Excellence and power in clinical nursing practice.* Menlo Park, CA: Addison-Wesley.

Dossey, B. M., Keegan, L., Kolkmeier, L. G., & Guzzetta, C. E. (Eds.). (1989). *Holistic health promotion: A guide for practice.* Rockville, MD: Aspen Publishers.

Erikson, E. H. (1963). *Childhood and society* (2nd ed., reissued with 1981 afterthought). New York: W.W. Norton.

Fitzpatrick, J. (1983). A life perspective rhythm model. In J. J. Fitzpatrick & A. L. Whall (Eds.), *Conceptual models of nursing: Analysis and application* (pp. 295–302). Bowie, MD: Robert J. Brady.

Hall, L. E. (1966). Another view of nursing care and quality. In K. M. Straub & K. S. Parker (Eds.), *Continuity of patient care: The role of nursing* (pp. 47–66). Washington, DC: Catholic University of America Press.

Johnson, D. E. (1980). The behavioral system model for nursing. In J. P. Riehl

& C. Roy (Eds.), *Conceptual models for nursing practice* (2nd ed., pp. 207–216). New York: Appleton-Century-Crofts.

King, I. M. (1981). *A theory for nursing: Systems, concepts, process.* New York: Wiley.

Leininger, M. M. (1991). The theory of culture care diversity and universality. In M. M. Leininger (Ed.), *Culture care diversity & universality: A theory of nursing* (pp. 5–68). New York: National League for Nursing.

Levine, M. E. (1971). Holistic nursing. *Nursing Clinics of North America, 2,* 253–264.

Longway, I. (1970). Toward a philosophy of nursing. *Journal of Adventist Education, 3,* 20–27.

Newman, M. A. (1986). *Health as expanding consciousness.* St. Louis, MO: C.V. Mosby.

Orem, D. E. (1985). *Nursing: Concepts of practice* (3rd ed.). New York: McGraw-Hill.

Orlando, I. J. (1990). *The dynamic nurse–patient relationship.* New York: National League for Nursing.

Quinn, J. F. (1992). Holding sacred space: The nurse as healing environment. *Holistic Nursing Practice, 4,* 26–36.

Rogers, M. E. (1970). *An introduction to the theoretical basis of nursing.* Philadelphia: F.A. Davis.

Rogers, M. E. (1990). Nursing: Science of unitary, irreducible, human beings: Update 1990. In E.A.M. Barrett (Ed.), *Visions of Rogers' science-based nursing* (pp. 1–11). New York: National League for Nursing.

Roy, C. (1980). The Roy adaptation model. In J. P. Riehl & C. Roy (Eds.), *Conceptual models for nursing practice* (2nd ed., pp. 179–188). New York: Appleton-Century-Crofts.

Rubin, R. (1968). A theory of clinical nursing. *Nursing Research, 3,* 210–212.

Scott, D. W., Oberst, M. T., & Dropkin, M. J. (1980). A stress-coping model. *Advances in Nursing Science, 1,* 9–24.

Watson, J. (1988). *Nursing: Human science and human care.* New York: National League for Nursing.

Whall, A, L. (1980). Congruence between existing theories of family functioning and nursing theories. *Advances in Nursing Science, 1,* 59–68.

Wilber, K. *(1980) The Atman project: A transpersonal view of human development.* Wheaton, IL: Theosophical Publishing House.

16 *Theories Focusing on the Nurse–Patient Relationship*

All theories must deal with nurse–patient relationships in some fashion, but there are several classes of theories that take the *interchange* as their focus. This chapter looks at two classes: the first, interaction theories; the second, those with an existential base.

INTERACTION THEORIES

Any theory that locates its principles in the nature of the exchange between the patient and the nurse is an *interaction theory*. Several well-known nursing theories take this stance. Although they share a focus on the relationship itself, they vary greatly in other ways. Take, for example, the radical difference between Orlando (1990) and Watson (1988)—Orlando, pragmatic, tied to what is observed and what it means; Watson, metaphysical, developmental, spiritual. Yet both theories rest their principles on the interplay between the two actors: patient and nurse.

INTERACTION COMMUNICATIONS MODELS

Orlando's (1990) theory is interactional because it depends on a particular ritualized back-and-forth dance between patient and nurse—a dance in which each party has his assigned role. The nurse observes the patient's behavior, interprets it, then reflects back to the patient what she has seen and what she thinks it means. The patient, in turn, reflects on the behavior, correcting errors, if any, in her interpretation, often gaining insight into behaviors not previously

Barbara J. Stevens Barnum: NURSING THEORY:
ANALYSIS, APPLICATION, EVALUATION, FOURTH EDITION.
© 1994, 1990, 1984, 1979 J.B. Lippincott.

brought to the forefront of his attention. Only after the nurse knows the meaning of the behavior as the patient sees it does she act on the behavior to solve the patient's problem. As Orlando (1990) has said, "Learning how to understand what is happening between herself and the patient is the central core of the nurse's practice and comprises the basic framework for the help she gives to patients." (p. 5)

As an interaction theory, Orlando's locates nursing in communication—verbal and behavioral—as do most older interaction theories. The vulnerability of these theories is that they are hard to apply to patients who cannot communicate (the unconscious, confused, or withdrawn).

King (1981) presents another theory that is a dance of roles between patient and nurse. In essence, her theory of nursing is built on a communications model in which patient and nurse mutually perceive, judge, act, react, interact, then mutually transact. As King described it,

> All behavior is communication that can be observed directly or indirectly. Experiences can be communicated from one person to another to build a common frame of reference. This can be called a reciprocally contingent interaction, which means that the behavior of patients is influenced by the behavior of nurses and vice versa. Transactions occur within systems of interactions of person with person, person with object, in which continuous motion and energy exchange is organized by information. When there is a disturbance in patterns of transactions, something has disrupted abilities to function, and individuals seek assistance. . . .
>
> Interactions are reciprocal. When one initiates an interaction with another, an action takes place, each person reacts to the other, and a reciprocal spiral develops in which the individuals continue to interact or withdraw from the situation. Each has something to give to the other that the other wants or needs, which may be facilitated by active participation of both individuals in the situation. There is a mutuality, an interdependence in the situation in which both achieve goals (pp. 82–84).

Both Orlando and King are vulnerable to the question of boundary, that is, they need to explain what context makes the interaction a nursing interaction as opposed to an interaction of another kind. Peplau, another nurse theorist with an interaction theory, has escaped this criticism by closely tying her middle-range theory to psychiatric nursing or psychotherapeutics in nursing. Peplau—whose works have been gathered and edited by O'Toole and Welt (1989)—has a goal-directed theory whose aim is to "help move the patient in a direction favoring productive social living outside of the hospital." (p. 197)

She described a patient's goal perception in the following manner:

> Psychiatric patients are embarked on a search for truth about themselves and their life experiences. This search is not for the literal, factual truths but rather for the inner truths about their perceptions and attributions of their experiences and the consequences in relationships with people. (Cited in O'Toole & Welt, 1989, p. 275)

She also identified the flaw that makes her interpersonal relations unidirectional in control (unlike King, who seems to stress reciprocity). For Peplau, the nurse is in command and sees it as her job not to let the conversation degenerate into social chitchat. But the method of conversation intimately involves both players. As Peplau (cited in O'Toole & Welt, 1989) said,

> Psychiatric patients are lacking the intellectual and interpersonal competencies so necessary for the work involved in their search for self-understanding. It is the quality of the verbal participation of nurses in their interactions with patients—listening and posing investigative questions—that slowly but surely stimulates the development of these competencies in patients (p. 275).

In essence, Peplau's nurse is an investigator, prober, interpreter, and reporter, using the rich data she extracts from the patient concerning his life. She develops insight (hers and his) into the meaning of a patient's behavior (including verbal behavior) and helps the patient recognize and change patterns that obstruct achievement of his goals.

Not that Peplau came right out and said this in her writings. Instead, she revealed her principles in demonstration, showing her process in individual cases that illustrated the effective nurse. She kept her cases related to psychiatric nursing, for example, nurse responses to unique patient cases of anxiety, frustration, withdrawal, loneliness, and aggression. Use of the case method allows her reader to gain insights through the "aha" method—a teaching technique that is often thought superior to merely spelling out one's principles.

In essence, all three authors, Orlando, King, and Peplau, have a *process* of interaction. Although Orlando and King apply theirs in situations in which nurses and patients meet, the content and context elements of their theories are not tightly defined. In essence, there are pieces of their theories that need more development. Peplau, on the other hand, has content and context pieces—phenomena located in psychiatric nursing.

INTERACTION MODELS IN NEW PARADIGM THEORIES

Although the content and context of new paradigm models have little in common with the interaction theories just discussed, they often share the focus on the unique nurse–patient interrelationship. Watson's (1988) theory illustrates the point. She asserted that "caring as an intersubjective human process is the moral ideal of nursing," (p. 39) and explained that

> the human care transactions provide a coming together and establishment of contact between persons; one's mind-body-soul engages with another's mind-body-soul in a lived moment. The shared moment of the present has the potential to transcend time and space and the physical, concrete world as we generally view it in the traditional nurse–patient relationship (p. 47).

Although the prior interaction theories envisioned a phenomenal nurse–patient relationship, Watson's theory envisions, instead, a transcendental one, a relationship "with the potential to transcend time and space"—nothing down to earth here. Depending on one's personal perspective, Watson's theory makes the others sound old fashioned, or, conversely, the others make hers sound frivolous and unrealistic. Notice how well these two perspectives—both interactional—illustrate the point that external criticism (how well a theory reflects the reality) is in the mind of the beholder. We turn next to another type of theory that focuses on the nurse–patient relationship: the existential theory.

EXISTENTIAL THEORIES

In Chapter 10, an *existential interpretation* was described as one in which the human agent's acts, ideas, or impulses are what characterizes the world. Acting within that interpretation, a whole school of philosophy—existentialism—emerged and held sway in the philosophic and public press more than three decades ago. Nursing also had its advocates in the movement. In nursing, the theorists who most closely represented this position were Paterson and Zderad (1988). They are included in this discussion because, even today, some schools follow their theory. More commonly, some elements of it are borrowed and tucked into other theories—often the emerging New Age developmental ones.

To understand what is unique about their theory, we start with a basic understanding of the themes and drives in existentialism. Existentialism, in the common parlance, is best understood through the themes that arise repeatedly and characterize the movement. Even given these central themes, there is little agreement as to who is and who is not an existentialist.

Dominant Themes in Existentialism

The term *existentialism* indicates that one begins with what exists—in this case, the human agent. (Any philosophy buffs will recognize that I lean heavily on the German existentialists for the interpretation that follows.) Existence precedes essence: the agent exists but what he becomes is not predetermined. There is no foreordained human nature. Man exists; his *being there* is the first reality about him. He is, as Heidegger (1962, pp. 78–90) said, thrown into the world. The existentialist starts with absurdity—that man simply is there (an absurdity because it does not relate to some other cause or explanation).

Furthermore, man is the only being who asks why he is there. A dog lives out his life without ever asking why he exists—but not man. Introspection, then, characterizes man; he not only exists but asks what it *means* to exist. He is concerned with the fact of his own existence.

Another tenet of existentialism is that, once he exists, man creates himself, that is, determines his own essence. The freedom to create and to choose is one of the major themes of existentialism. One chooses, and what one chooses determines what one becomes. One literally makes himself through his choices. Because choosing is an ongoing necessity, man is never a finished product; he is always in the state of becoming.

Although existentialism escapes the fatalism of a deterministic philosophy (in which every act is preordained by what preceded it), the freedom it espouses is not without its price. The existentialist cannot blame today's bad choice on yesterday's events; he is fully responsible for each choice he makes. Although the past is determined (it cannot be changed), the future is open to any possibility (Sartre, 1965, pp. 409–532). Hence, time is experienced as "the present toward the future."

To choose is a freedom that some perceive as a burden. Some choices, for example, must be made repeatedly. A dieter decides anew every time he passes the refrigerator. A marriage vow must be confirmed again every time an opportunity to negate it arises. The need to decide in the ongoing present (and the responsibility for the decision) are central themes in existentialism. Choices once made are irrevocable; one cannot turn back the clock to undo a decision.

One cannot ever again be the person he was before a particular decision was made. The past is fixed, and he is responsible for it. The future is open to whatever choices he makes.

It also is impossible to choose with knowledge. One cannot debate: if I make Choice X, I will become this type of person, but if I make Choice Y, I will become that sort. Decision making is not grounded in knowledge. On the contrary, knowledge is the result of decision making and subsequent action. It is not possible to predict with certainty; so one makes choices and thereby chooses oneself without knowing the result.

The need to choose in the light of uncertainty calls for a leap into the unknown, and for this reason, many existentialists associate choice with dread, anxiety, or despair (Kierkegaard, 1954, pp. 147–207). Other philosophers delight in the creativity and power of such ultimate freedom, celebrating, instead of dreading, those leaps into the unknown.

Because *choice* is what constitutes man, to choose in light of the unknown represents an authentic, honest mode of being. Avoidance of choice and escapism of various sorts represent inauthentic modes of being—being as *nonbeing*. Nonbeing is an alienation from oneself; authenticity is a major virtue.

Failure to accept responsibility for the results of one's choices is *inauthentic* being. One acts and is accountable. Denial of one's emotions also is a form of inauthenticity; to negate one's feelings is dishonest because it denies one's experiences.

The existential philosophy has little room for intentions; what counts is acts performed, not acts—or results—intended. One is what one does; acts define the self. Potentialities do not count.

Because the results of leaps into the unknown, occasioned by choices, cannot be predicted rationally, the existential philosophy is based on examination of passions rather than reason. Feeling is concrete, particular, immediate, and subjective; in contrast, thinking is universal, abstract, removed from immediacy, and objective. Suffering often is posited as the origin of consciousness in existentialism. Awareness of self does not arise through thought. Theories do not give us reality; reality must be experienced.

Many (but not all) philosophers who are classified as existentialists share the following six dominant themes:

1. Man exists as being-in-the-world, and his existence precedes his essence (what he becomes).
2. Freedom and choice characterize man.
3. Man forms himself through his choices.
4. Freedom may be seen as terrible and burdensome or as a joy.

5. Emotion and passion characterize man better than does reason.
6. The individual (not the society or group) is the proper unit of analysis.

Nature of the Self in Existentialism

In existentialism, the quest is for understanding of self and what it means to be a self. Many writers have proposed that a self has the following five characteristics:

1. The self feels unfinished, incomplete; he exists as an open being, always becoming, never finished.
2. The self does not experience a mind–body split but feels himself to be a whole.
3. The self perceives himself as a unity, despite having many selves with which to fill the many different roles of day-to-day life.
4. Although he may change radically over time, man perceives himself as an ongoing unit; he has a sense of a continuing *me*.
5. The nature of that *me*, extracted from the content with which it deals, is problematic; motion or drive may be its chief characteristic.

The search for understanding of self (that which is conscious of its own being) is critical in existential thought. The source of knowledge is a close examination of one's own feelings, responses, and awareness of being. Evidence is not of the analytical sort found in scientific research.

Existential Relationships

Existentialists differ on the nature of the relationship between self and other. Some have claimed that only knowledge of the self is possible, that the other is merely an object for the self. Other theorists have argued that if one accepts the reality of being for oneself, then one must grant it for others.

Many existentialists focus on man's intersubjectivity, exploring the nature of *genuine encounter*. (This is where the existential philosophy enters into the theories based on the nurse–patient relationship.) Typically, an authentic encounter is seen as one in which each person reveals his authentic being to the other and in which each person is able to grasp the reality of the other person.

EXISTENTIAL APPLICATIONS IN NURSING

The initial attraction of existentialism for nurses could be accounted for by the apparent fit of the existential reality with the nursing environment. Because authentic relationships occur one-to-one, the format is natural for nursing. Furthermore, the nurse finds herself in an environment in which she and the dyadic other are exposed to strong emotions, questions concerning self-worth, and even fears for the continued existence of the self. Moreover, the situation demands that the nurse face constant choices (often critical) in providing care.

Sister Vaillot (1962) described the existential environment in relation to student nurses:

> They see people grieve, suffer, or rejoice with an intensity that seems hardly possible for humans to bear. They see women give birth, and they see patients die. They see men and women in such crises that they are stripped naked of what they have: wealth, prestige, beauty, status, intelligence, and only the person that they really are is left. Student nurses are, almost every minute of their professional life, confronted with the choice between acceptance and refusal of these situation-limits. They can be a presence to patients, and follow the road leading to authentic being (p. 42).

Vaillot also indicated the predominance of emotive force (commitment) over reason:

> No nurse can find personal fulfillment in her chosen occupation, nor ensure the growth and the social usefulness of nursing, unless she is committed to it. One of the basic tasks facing nurse educators, then, is to find ways of fostering commitment on the part of their students (p. 25).

Notice that commitment is her key word, not knowledge. Jourard (1971) stayed in the emotive vein but focused on the evolving self of the nurse as it relates to potentiality for nursing others:

> The becoming general nursing practitioner is a person who is open to her own experience, who genuinely cares about people and about herself. This is important. She cares about herself. The proof of effective caring about oneself is a self which is happy, growing, open (p. 284).

Jourard contrasted this sort of personal growth and becoming with education, efficiency, and effortlessness, and asserted that these traits (often associated with professionalism) may actively obstruct growth (p. 285). Again, the existential focus is on authenticity, not cognition.

Sarosi (1968) also described nursing in existential terms:

> Nursing action, then, is affirmation and validation of human experience, and is characterized by involvement, not composure or "objectivity." The desired outcome is wholeness, not comfort (p. 353).

Realization of uniqueness, of human finiteness, may be experienced by the individual through his encounter with death and loneliness. Thus loneliness and death must be confronted rather than escaped from. It is this encounter which leads man to the infinite, to an awareness of "the inseparability of his organism from the cosmos. Existence is relationship; to be is to be related." (p. 356)

The classic existential nurse theorists are Paterson and Zderad (1988); not surprisingly, they focused on the nurse–patient relationship. The flavor of their work together can be sensed in the following quotations:

Nurses experience with other human beings peak life events: creation, birth, winning, nothingness, losing, separation, death. . . . Through in-touchness with self, authentic awareness and reflection on such experiences the human nurse comes to know. Humanistic nursing practice theory asks that the nurse describe what she comes to know: (1) the nurse's unique perspective and responses, (2) the other's knowable responses, and (3) the reciprocal call and response, the between, as they occur in the nursing situation (pp. 6–7).

Notice the focus on awareness and authenticity and on the emotional, experiential aspects of nursing. These all demonstrate the existential focus. The next quotation not only reveals their existential base but shows why existential nursing theories find their principle in relationships:

In real life, nursing phenomena may be experienced from the reference points of nurturing, of being nurtured, or of the nurturing process in the "between." For instance, the nurse may describe comfort as an experience of comforting another person; the patient, as an experience of being comforted. However, while each has experienced something within himself, he also has experienced something of the "between," namely the message of meaning of the "comforting-being comforted" process. This essential interhuman dimension of nursing is beyond and yet within the technical, procedural, or interactional elements of the event. It is a quality of being that is expressed in the doing (Paterson & Zderad, 1988, p. 13).

Notice how the older existentialist language resembles the language of some theorists in the New Age paradigm. It is true, the themes sound similar, but the context is quite different. Existentialists deal with phenomenal experience—what is seen, felt—directly. In contrast, the New Agers seek transcendental explanations for events—in phenomena such as energy exchanges, resonating waves, human fields. Although there are religious existentialists, they are usually in mainstream religious orthodoxy. In contrast, the New Agers usually express man's spirituality as a development toward higher levels of being in which man participates in an ultimate conscious unity.

Despite these differences, the flavor of these two movements (existentialism and New Ageism) is similar, particularly the great human sensitivity for the other and the self. Both nursing philosophies focus on the one-to-one human relationship as the vehicle through which nursing occurs.

The nurse theorist who advocates an existential approach must ask serious questions concerning the nature of nursing. If an existential interpretation is merely an overlay, not actually impacting on what the nurse does as a nurse, then it is not an inherent part of a nursing theory. It is not enough to advocate an existential approach in nursing; one must say how it changes the day-to-day acts of nurses.

When an existential approach is used to explain nurse behavior that could occur under any other nursing philosophy, then the application is superficial. The existential goal (authentic being), for example, may be incompatible with some well-accepted, traditional nursing goals. Does the nurse remain true to the existential values despite the professional norms?

The approach to the patient in pain illustrates the potential conflict. From an existential viewpoint, suffering serves to bring about a state of self-awareness, thereby creating an openness to authentic experience. Suffering brings a person face to face with his own being. Yet most nurses would seek to alleviate suffering rather than prolong it as an instrument of self-realization. A nurse who purports to use an existential theory must be prepared to deal with such challenges. Similarly, the skills of communication taught to nurses often are manipulative devices designed to achieve certain ends—possibly worthy ends—but not the end of genuine intersubjectivity. The issue of manipulation (obviously inauthentic being—treating the other as an object) must be handled in a truly existential nursing theory.

Then there is the issue of genuine encounter. Because most existentialists consider genuine encounter to be an experience that shakes one's self-world, one need ask how many such encounters a nurse could be expected to endure. A nurse–patient relationship arises in every patient-care assignment, but can genuine encounters be assigned? Furthermore, genuine encounters are two-way interactions, and some patients may not wish to play the game.

One might argue that in an era in which so many illnesses are related to life-style, an existential approach holds interesting promise. But about the only place one sees it used today is in some substance abuse programs. Unlike the Alcoholics Anonymous programs that treat alcoholism as a disease, some confrontational programs attempt to administer a reality shock by placing blame and challenging the patient to accept responsibility for his own conduct.

The Toughlove program for parents of substance abusing youths has a similar confrontational theme.

In summary, existential theories of nursing, probably best represented by Paterson and Zderad, appear to have been upstaged by theories focused in a New Age paradigm. Yet one can see some similarities in tone. Compare, for example, Paterson and Zderad's (1988, pp. 27–29) notion of the nurse as *presence* with Quinn's (1992) notion of the nurse as a sacred place, a healing environment. Parse (1981) is probably the best example of the crossover from existentialism to New Ageism. Indeed, one could argue that she still sits on the fence between the two ideologies. Take, for example, her assumptions, which she admittedly draws from Heidegger (1962), Merleau-Ponty (1962), and Sartre (1965) (all existentialists) as well as Rogers (1990), whose work certainly was instrumental in initiating New Ageism in nursing. Parse's (1981) assumptions—rearranged for this purpose—include, but are not limited to, the following:

- Man is an open being, freely choosing meaning in situation, bearing responsibility for decisions.
- Health is an open process of becoming, experienced by man.
- Man is transcending multidimensionality with the possibles.
- Health is unitary man's negentropic unfolding (p. 25).

If the first two assumptions smack of existentialism, the last two are soundly grounded in the New Age paradigm.

It may be the fact that existential and New Age philosophies focus on the nurse–patient interrelationship that makes them bedfellows. They certainly share a poetry of tone and sentiment that is not found in the interaction theories of King, Peplau, and Orlando, for example. Yet there is a great difference between an existentialist and an advocate of a New Age paradigm. In essence, the existentialists accept the absurdity of man's existence, whereas the New Agers do not find it absurd or pointless at all.

SUMMARY

There are several types of nursing theory that revolve around the nurse–patient interaction. Often this is the only similarity they bear. Older interactions models tend to focus on a communications model that is based heavily on interpersonal communication. King, Peplau, and Orlando represent this trend. Their age is not the measure of their use in the profession, and all three models are still used today.

Newer interaction models occur in the New Age paradigm, but here the notion of communication has expanded to encompass much more than verbal communication. Notions of mind–body–soul engagement between patient and nurse or of therapeutic touch illustrate these larger notions of communication.

Existential theories of authentic encounter also are found under the category of nurse–patient interaction. These older theories often have been replaced by New Age paradigm images or melded with ideas arising in this new context. Whatever the source, theories based on the nurse–patient interaction place their principles in the critical juncture between two people rather than in one or the other.

REFERENCES

Heidegger, M. (1962). *Being and time* (J. Macquarrie & E. Robinson, Trans.). New York: Harper & Row.

Jourard, S. (1971). *The transparent self.* New York: Van Nostrand Reinhold.

Kierkegaard, S. (1954). *The sickness unto death* (W. Lowrie, Trans.). Garden City, NY: Doubleday.

King, I. M. (1981). *A theory for nursing: Systems, concepts, process.* New York: Wiley.

Merleau-Ponty, M. (1962). *Phenomenology of perception.* New York: Humanities Press.

Orlando, I. J. (1990). *The dynamic nurse–patient relationship.* New York: National League for Nursing.

O'Toole, A. W., & Welt, S. R. (Eds.). (1989). *Interpersonal theory in nursing practice: Selected works of Hildegard E. Peplau.* New York: Springer.

Parse, R. R. (1981). *Man–living–health: A theory of nursing.* New York: Wiley.

Paterson, J. G., & Zderad, L. T. (1988). *Humanistic nursing.* New York: National League for Nursing.

Quinn, J. F. (1992). Holding sacred space: The nurse as healing environment. *Holistic Nursing Practice, 4,* 26–36.

Rogers, M. E. (1990). Nursing: Science of unitary, irreducible, human beings: Update 1990. In E. A. M. Barrett (Ed.) *Visions of Rogers' science-based nursing* (pp. 5–11) New York: National League for Nursing.

Sarosi, G. M. (1968). A critical theory: The nurse as a fully human person. *Nursing Forum, 4,* 349–364.

Sartre, J. P. (1965). *Being and nothingness* (H. E. Barnes, Trans.). New York: Citadel Press.

Vaillot, M. C. (1962). *Commitment to nursing: A philosophic investigation.* Philadelphia: J. B. Lippincott.

Watson, J. (1988). *Nursing: Human science and human care: A theory of nursing.* New York: National League for Nursing.

BIBLIOGRAPHY

Bergson, H. (1911). *Matter and memory.* New York: Macmillan.

Gulino, C. K. (1982). Entering the mysterious dimension of other: An existential approach to nursing care. *Nursing Outlook, 6,* 352–357.

Marcel, G. (1950). *The mystery of being.* Chicago: Regnery Press.

May, R. (1958). *Existence: A new dimension in psychiatry and psychology.* New York: Basic Books.

Merleau-Ponty, M. (1963). *The structure of behavior.* Boston: Beacon Press.

Riceour, P. (1965). *Fallible man.* Chicago: Regnery Press.

Sartre, J. P. (1957). *Transcendence of the ego.* New York: Noonday Press.

17 Resource-Driven Nursing: A Model for Practice and Management

PRACTICE MODELS

Nurses have struggled valiantly to adjust to increasingly difficult work situations. In many cases, they simply have had to lower their expectations concerning what could be accomplished for patients. An adjustment to scarcities of staff and proper supplies and equipment, despite increasing patient acuity, has been the rule, not the exception. Many nurses have developed a sense of general dissatisfaction with their roles, not to mention disillusion with the health care system.

Nowhere has the difference between expectations and realities been greater than in the acute care facility. We will use this setting for the following discussion, although the principles derived can be applied in any setting.

Total Patient Care

Let us start with a review of some favorite notions of nursing care from the past. Total patient care—comprehensive nursing care, if you prefer—used to be the order of the day. The assumption was that the nurse would provide "everything" for the patients assigned to her. There was no notion of compromise, of limitations, no sense that a patient was only paying for X amount of care. A whole generation of nurses was educated on this model.

But the model of total patient care was designed to work in ideal conditions. And a model made for ideal conditions is vulnerable

Barbara J. Stevens Barnum: NURSING THEORY:
ANALYSIS, APPLICATION, EVALUATION, FOURTH EDITION.
© 1994, 1990, 1984, 1979 J.B. Lippincott.

when nurses cannot produce those conditions. That is what has happened today: many nurses still hold themselves accountable for standards they cannot achieve. Worse, these nurses place their notion of self-worth in the comprehensiveness of their care for each patient. If they cannot do "everything" needed, they judge themselves to be failures.

Notice that the concept of *total patient care* was based on abstract, idealistic goals. No constraints were to be considered; the nurse was limited in identifying patient needs only by her own intellectual capacities. She was responsible for providing everything that was deemed to be good for the patient. In this respect, total patient care was a *goal-driven* model (Barnum & Mallard, 1989, pp. 35–42). A nurse could not claim success unless she identified all the potential patient needs, set all the possible goals, and met them.

In recent years, total nursing care (goal-driven care) has been impossible in many places, and nurses have been forced to compromise. A makeshift sort of care has evolved, a care pattern that might be called *doing what one could*. This is another case in which a practice arose before it had been framed in theoretical terms. The rest of this chapter attempts to provide a theoretical structure that both reflects the practice (doing what one could) and, more important, sets forth the dimensions of a model so that nurses can use it effectively rather than fumbling through without a plan.

The Resource-Driven Model

In contrast to the goal-driven care of yesterday, the care going on today should be labeled *resource-driven* care. In a resource-driven model, the nurse first considers her environment and the resources it holds. Only then does she determine what goals she reasonably can take on for a group of patients. The resources drive the goals, not the other way around. This is the opposite of the total patient care concept, in which goals are set first, assuming that the necessary resources will be found.

Resource-driven care stands the old model on its head, and that hits hard at a philosophy of care most nurses hold dear. It is particularly hard for a nurse who has been indoctrinated to think that her worth is tied to doing "everything" for her patients. It calls for a new outlook, a new measure on which to gage one's worth.

A resource-driven model also is more complex than a goal-driven model. It demands more choices, a more accurate fit between available resources and the work to be done. If total patient care took its origin in quality factors of good care, then resource-driven care demands a mesh of quality and quantity (how much care at what quality).

The most important quantity factor in the new system is the nurse's own work time. The question becomes how much and what sort of care she can deliver in a limited number of hours. Other resources may expand, but one never gets more than 24 hours in a day. True, a nurse may compensate by working overtime (usually without compensation), but she will find that she can only subsidize the system so long before she is mentally and physically bankrupt.

Many nurses remember school days, when they could take hours in the library to complete a nursing care plan for a single patient. The nurse did not have to make any hard choices. She poured everything into that care plan, being careful not to skip a single goal that might help the patient.

Resource-driven care has not that luxury. Today's nurse seldom has just one patient. Often she must balance the needs of a group of patients considered together. She must make much more complex professional decisions—determining what things she will do for which patients, knowing that her priorities are critical and that she must often make hard choices between the essential and the merely beneficial. Indeed, the resource-driven model is a triage model not unlike that used in emergency room or disaster nursing.

COMPARISON OF SYSTEMS

The easiest way to understand a resource-driven model of care is to compare it with the goal-driven model. There are numerous dimensions on which they differ.

The first dimension has to do with underlying assumptions. For the goal-driven model, it was assumed that all worthy goals would be tackled. With initiative, the nurse would find the necessary resources, including the requisite time.

The resource-driven model has no such optimism. It assumes that the nurse's time is finite and so is her access to additional resources. Instead, she must plan within the constraints of available manpower, supplies, and equipment in the institution. These items are unlikely to expand simply because she can identify a need for them.

The process of planning patient care is accordingly quite different in the two models. In the goal-driven model, it goes like this: The nurse sets goals based on the patient's case description or her own assessments. When she has set all the desirable goals she can determine, she decides on the methods (interventions) to achieve the goals. Next, she implements the methods. Finally, she evaluates whether the goals have been achieved.

The process in the resource-driven model is more complex. The nurse begins not with an assessment of the patient, but with an assessment of the resources at hand. How many hours will she work? What staff, if any, are assigned to assist her? What sorts of support are available? Whereas the goal-directed nurse started with a quality issue (the patient's needs and goals), this nurse starts with a quantity assessment of resources—man-hours available being the most important single calculation. Like the other nurse, the resource-directed nurse then assesses the patient as to his needs and calculates potential goals for his care.

From here, the picture gets more complicated. In the first place, one patient's care cannot be calculated alone—unless he comprises the nurse's full assignment. Instead, she considers as a whole the needs and potential goals for the whole caseload of patients. Next she starts the task of prioritizing—deciding what *must* be done, what is less critical. From the start, she works with a realization that not "everything" is likely to be achieved. Now she must match her priorities to the available resources. For simplicity, just consider the chief resource: her own time.

The resource-directed nurse cannot go directly from prioritized goals to an estimation of time required, because the time required may depend on the methods she selects to meet those goals. The interim step, then, requires that goals be considered in relation to alternate means of achieving them. For many goals, there may be some methods that are to be preferred (in the abstract) and others that may be less adequate but take less time and fewer resources.

Here, a subtle dance of professional judgment occurs. What goals can she meet, using what methods, all within the constraints of her resources? Notice how much simpler it was for the goal-directed nurse. All she had to do was "everything"; she did not have to make any hard choices. The nurse using the resource-driven model must be a more competent professional to make the best calculations, the best plans of care for all. In this situation, the nurse who says, "I was too busy to practice professionally today" misses the whole point. Hard choices call for sophisticated professional decisions.

Like the planning, the evaluation process is more complex in the resource-driven model. The nurse using a goal-driven model only needed to ask if she had achieved her goals. The nurse using the resource-driven model must make a lot more judgments:

- Did she make an *accurate* assessment of resources? Were there resources available that she failed to consider? Or did she overestimate her available time or the assistance she could call on?

- Did she take on an appropriate *number* of goals? Did she bite off too much, too little?
- Did she take on the *most important* goals? Or did she skip something that should have had a higher priority? Did she waste time on some goals that were impossible to achieve?
- Did she choose the best methods, considering the circumstances? Were there more efficient systems available? Were the methods effective?
- Did she achieve the goals selected? In this element, she comes back to the only evaluation item required on the goal-driven system.

LIMITATIONS AND ADVANTAGES OF BOTH SYSTEMS

What are the limitations of the two systems? The goal-driven system breaks down if the assumed resources cannot be found. For example, if the nurse simply does not have the time she anticipates, then she cannot achieve all her goals. Worse, because she may not realize the deficit until well into her shift, the things that get done and the things that get omitted may be unrelated to their importance. If the goal-driven system lacks the anticipated resources, the nurse has no recourse but to feel like a failure.

The resource-driven model has its limitations, too. It calls for more sophisticated practice if the right decisions are to be made. It is not a system for an amateur. Additionally, the resource-driven model requires a safety net. That means criteria must be set for recognizing when scarce resources are reaching the level of unsafe care. This is done by setting nursing standards and identifying indices that will quickly signal a dangerous situation. In simple terms, one index might be that of the lowest acceptable nurse–patient ratio. Criteria for recognizing a critical situation and plans for how to deal with the contingency should be set *in advance* of such a situation occurring.

What are the advantages of each system? The goal-driven system has the charm of allowing the nurse to practice at the peak of her performance and assure the patient of the best possible outcomes. Furthermore, the nursing process and its evaluation are comparatively simple, allowing less experienced nurses to achieve success with minimal stress.

The resource-driven model, in contrast, has the advantage of adapting to its environment when it is not within the nurse's power to change it. In a resource-scarce environment, this can be a distinct advantage. Furthermore, a nurse working in such circumstances can still feel satisfied with her performance. In essence, she can say to herself, "Given the circumstances, I made the best choices possible, did the most and most effective work that could be done."

Interestingly, the resource-driven model also works in a *resource-rich* environment. When the nurse calculates what can be done in this case, she will find herself able to take on a plethora of goals.

ADDITIONAL THOUGHTS

Advocates of the resource-driven model would assert that excellence in nursing practice has never truly been separate from environmental conditions. Excellent nursing, such advocates would say, can occur in the most difficult of circumstances. Nightingale started a profession in Crimea despite her bleak surroundings (or because of her bleak surroundings, some would say). Excellence is optimizing on the possible; simply put, it is what one does with what one has got.

The question is one of the nurse's assumed power to change an environment. The goal-driven model assumes she can do so to an extent encompassing the best of all worlds. The resource-driven model is more realistic, recognizing that not all of the negative factors within the environment are within her control.

The resource-driven model asks how well the nurse did in the circumstances, not how well she did in the abstract. Nurses educated on a model of the ideal may be uncomfortable with this model initially, but it builds a new standard for judging one's worth.

MANAGEMENT MODELS

With management models, we find a situation that corresponds directly to what we found in the care-delivery models. Just as a resource-driven model is replacing a goal-driven model in nursing care, so a resource-driven model is replacing a goal-driven model in management.

The older model, management by objectives (MBO), is clearly a goal-driven model—just look at its name. The pattern is identical to goal-driven nursing care: first you set the goals, then you find the resources.

Strategic Management

MBO is rapidly being replaced by a strategic management model (Barnum & Mallard, 1989, pp. 66–69). Strategic management starts by assessing the environment—internal to the organization and external to it. It assesses the organization's strengths and weaknesses in comparison with those of the competition. This marketplace mentality, tied as it is to environmental conditions, parallels the resource-driven care model.

Only after the environment is carefully scanned and assessed will goals be selected in the strategic management model. Goals will be those that can reasonably be taken on, given environmental constraints, or those that optimize opportunities. As with the resource-driven model, the focus is on choosing the right actions. The effective organization is the one that makes the most advantageous choices, based on the most accurate assessment of the environment.

In strategic planning, not only is the management scheme designed with the environment in mind, but it is made flexible to change as the external environment changes. Quick response is more important than the old 2-year and 5-year plans of MBO. Assessment, of necessity, becomes ongoing rather than periodic.

In strategic management, the image is moving, swift, changing—not at all like MBO, in which one assumes that most elements are in one's control. In strategic planning, like the resource-driven care model, the outside world impinges on and affects one's plans.

Strategic planning involves drawing up alternate scenarios, alternate plans designed for meeting different environmental contingencies. The strategic plan lacks the stability and security of the MBO model; it is not a simple rational plan.

The vulnerability of MBO management is its assumption that one *can* plan ahead. It assumes a stable, unchanging world, in which one can set goals that will still be appropriate 1 year, 2 years, or 5 years later. In a world changing as fast as today's health care, such an assumption does not have a chance.

Mintzberg's Models

Mintzberg (1973) anticipated the changing models of management two decades ago when he wrote about three managerial styles: (1) the rational planning, (2) adaptive, and (3) entrepreneurial modes. His rational-planning model sounded perfect then; it typified the MBO approach in which advance planning was done. The system seemed ideal in a world in which the effects of actions could be predicted and anticipated to hold over long time spans. Nurses wrote in praise of the model then, not inaccurately labeling it *proactive* instead of *reactive*.

From today's perspective, however, the other two models make more sense. The entrepreneurial mode allows the high risk taker, who has just a bit more vision or predictive power than the rest, to make her mark in an uncertain world. She takes bold strokes—and wins or loses accordingly. This form of management has great possibilities in our world in which so many unexpected changes can happen overnight. The environment is indeed ripe for the ambitious, clever entrepreneur.

Most management, certainly most health care management, presently focuses on the adaptive model instead of the entrepreneurial model. Strategic planning epitomizes this view with its constant reassessment of the environment and its rapid response to changes.

Strategic management is not the only new model around. In nursing management, as in other management systems, one sees the adoption of a new concept called *futures management,* an ideology that tries to have the best of both the goal-driven and resource-driven models. Preferred futures management, like strategic planning, envisions various future scenarios. Then, like the goal-driven model, selects the preferred scenario (i.e., setting goals).

Next the model switches back to the action-oriented strategic management approach—or better yet, to the entrepreneurial model—because the manager takes the bold strides to try to bring about that preferred future (Anvaripour, Bezold, & Weissman, 1990). Choosing a preferred future and making it happen is quite different from the *forecasting* advocated in the MBO model. In the MBO notion, the future is externally imposed; one strives to predict it, not create it.

LEADERSHIP AND THE TRANSFORMATIONAL LEADER

Not only do the new management models reflect the nature of the times, so do the images of the manager. In the era of MBO, the leader was contrasted with the manager, and the manager usually came out ahead. A manager could be trained, educated; the process was logical. This was more to be desired than spontaneous and uncontrolled leadership.

Now, in an era when the future is difficult to predict, when the environment is characterized by frequent, unpredictable changes, the notion of leadership once again has superseded the notion of the rational manager. The latest notion in the nursing literature (as well as the business literature) is the transformational leader.

The change is from what the leader *does* to who the leader *is* and how she motivates those who are led. Unlike the prior management ideology, transformational leadership assumes that the leader and followers have the same purpose, that they can raise one another to higher levels of motivation and morality. This notion certainly has appeal when both leader and followers are professionals.

The notion of transformational leadership is often tied to the New Age paradigm (Barker, 1991). She has asserted that a new view of humanness is emerging, that people are bringing to the workplace a new set of beliefs and values. The old paradigm, in contrast, focused on logical decision making, rationality.

Transformational leadership is essentially more human, with the leader seeking a new set of values emerging between herself and her workers: mutual cooperation instead of competition, attention to human needs and feelings, consultative interactions instead of downward-directed orders from the hierarchy, and empowerment of all employees, not just the chief.

Transformational leaders, so goes the theory, mobilize others; they grow and develop together with their followers. As one set of needs and values are satisfied for all parties, new ones surface and contribute to personal and professional growth.

It is easy to see the results of transformational leadership, because it shows in a focus on goals, joy in work, enthusiasm about patients and the care they receive, and a sense of accomplishment shared by all. Notice how these characteristics differ from the sort of talk one hears under an MBO ideology, that is, quotas, specified outcomes, measurement, data—cold, hard, incontrovertible facts.

The strategies used by a transformational leader involve

- creating a vision
- building a social architecture that shows how that vision will be institutionalized
- sustaining organizational trust
- recognizing the importance of building self-esteem (Barker, 1991, pp. 206–207).

Two polarities have always been used in looking at leadership: (1) whether the focus is on the leader or the followers and, (2) when the leader is the focus, whether the stress is on what she *does* or who she *is*. An MBO orientation focuses on what the leader does. Transformational leadership stresses who she is. Yet it also gives the followers more credence, because the response of the followers is the measure of the transformational leader's effectiveness.

SUMMARY

In a world of uncertainty, scarce resources, and increased competition, it is not surprising that our theoretical models are changing to reflect an altered environment. Perhaps the most interesting thing is how models for patient care, nursing management, and nurse manager behavior have all changed at the same time, all in ways that make them more compatible with today's health care environment.

As we saw with the nursing process, practices often are established before the models are neatly described and labeled as theories. The logic of these present changes should give us faith in the ultimate wit of man.

REFERENCES

Anvaripour, P., Bezold, C., & Weissman, G. (1990). A nursing department can and should plan for the future. Nursing & Health Care, 4, 207–209.

Barker, A. M. (1991). An emerging leadership pattern: Transformational leadership. Nursing & Health Care, 4, 204–207.

Barnum, B. S., & Mallard, C. O. (1989). Essentials of nursing management; Concepts and contest of practice. Rockville, MD: Aspen Publishers.

Mintzberg, H. (1973). Strategy making in three modes. California Management Review, 2, 44–53.

18 Nursing Theory and Restructured Practice

Nursing theory has always affected practice assignment systems, even in eras before theory was recognized as such. But theory alone is inadequate to explain the work delegation systems. The environmental circumstances also push and pull the choices. The present era has seen a radical change, namely the introduction of restructured nursing practice. We will explore this change from the dual perspectives of theory and circumstance.

If it has not already done so, virtually every major health delivery institution is presently restructuring its care delivery, and no two institutions are revising in just the same pattern. What the institutions share is the goal of restructured practice. Driven by economics, they all hope to improve or retain patient care capacity, given shrinking resources. Namely, they hope to optimize on the use of scarce professional nursing staff.

In an industry in which discretionary funds are highly limited, it was predictable that the recent welcome increases in nursing salaries would—sooner or later—demand a decrease in nursing staffing numbers. We see a circle of effects that could have been predicted:

- a shortage of nurses to meet the increasing demands of a health care industry in which patients are increasingly sicker, requiring more and more care
- enhancement of nursing as a career by increased salaries for nurses at all levels
- subsequent financial crises calling for decreases in professional staffing.

Ironically, the shortage that started the cycle has been solved not by eliminating the need for nurses, but by learning to live with

*Barbara J. Stevens Barnum: NURSING THEORY;
ANALYSIS, APPLICATION, EVALUATION, FOURTH EDITION.
© 1994, 1990, 1984, 1979 J.B. Lippincott.*

an unmet demand for care and by passing nursing tasks downward to less-skilled workers. In essence, the shortage has been met by eliminating positions from the marketplace. Now we will look at how this circumstance brought restructured practice into being.

DESCRIPTIONS

What is *restructured practice?* How does it manage the scarcity of professional nurses? Restructuring involves a careful analysis of the tasks that must be accomplished to deliver patient care and to achieve desired patient goals, along with an assessment of who is able to do the tasks.

Often in looking at who can do what, new jobs are created with new constellations of skills and educational qualifications. The decisions involve looking anew at the premises of prior task assignment decisions. Typically, restructured practice involves adding one or more levels of employees to the lower end of the care personnel rung, and moving tasks once seen as sacrosanct professional nursing turf down to lower-level workers.

The main principle underlying restructuring is not using overqualified personnel for tasks that can be achieved by less-skilled personnel. In many instances, this means creating new roles and combining tasks that may not have been previously joined under a single job description.

Although restructured practice is the terminology most often used, the linked term *differentiated practice* has come to mean almost the same thing. The demand for differentiated practice was first heard from nurse educators, and consisted of a demand that practice settings cease using all nurses as if they were alike. It was a demand that nurses be used differentially, based on their educational credentials.

Leaders who demanded differentiated practice envisioned that the baccalaureate-prepared nurse would have a different, more advanced role than nurses prepared in diploma and associate degree programs. One could say that the proponents of differentiated practice had their eyes on an upward movement for baccalaureate-prepared nurses.

Ironically, restructured practice gave them what they wanted—a system that differentiates roles according to preparation—but the view was downward, not upward. And most of the differentiation was between nurse and less well-prepared caregivers rather than between the baccalaureate-prepared nurse and nurses prepared in associate degree and diploma programs. Nevertheless, from a theoretical perspective, the same principle was at work: task distribution according to one's abilities, each employee used to the peak of his capacity.

THE HISTORICAL PERSPECTIVE

One of the easiest ways to understand restructured practice as a theory is to look at its place relevant to other historical shifts in nursing assignment systems. The pattern, from the long view, is dialectic—that is, there is a clear pattern of thesis, antithesis, and synthesis. In essence, a new assignment system always is in opposition to the system it replaces. The new system comes into being just when the flaws of the prior system have reached peak irritation. Then a contradictory pattern comes along to cure the flaws.

After an initial flurry of enthusiasm, the new pattern settles in and becomes the norm. Then, in time, its own limitations become onerous. A third pattern then emerges that combines the best traits of the prior systems but eliminates the most irritating aspects of the most recent one. With time, of course, another system comes along to challenge this one—and the pattern continues.

What brings an irritation to the forefront? In some cases, it can be blamed on familiarity, simply the test of time. In other cases, the environment impacts on the assignment system changes, making the flaw more obvious. In the recent shift to restructured practice, an altered environment forced a new system into existence. Chief among the changes was that institutions could no longer afford to hire all the nurses required for patients' care needs.

Let us look more closely at the history of assignment systems in the United States to get a sense of how a shift occurs. In this nation, even nursing in hospitals began with a *private duty* nursing model. The old private duty nurse had exclusive responsibility for planning for and doing for one patient. In this sense, private duty was a highly patient-oriented system. The nurse's role included around-the-clock care duties with few days off. Often she slept on a cot in the patient's hospital room—not unlike the system for nursing in the home.

That pattern began to rub because of an environmental change: a war, with nurses marching off to tend to the troops. In the subsequent civilian shortage of nurses, so-called *functional nursing* was conceived. As expected, it was the antithesis of the private duty model.

Functional nursing was driven by a need to improve the efficiency, to get more mileage from the few nurses available. The essential step was to shift from a *patient-based* system to a *task-based* system. This was done by the simple expedient of giving the hospital nurse tasks rather than patients.

In its day, functional nursing was hailed as a great invention.

As enacted then, functional nursing was a simple division of tasks according to ability or expertise. Instead of each nurse doing everything for one patient, tasks for patients on a unit were divided on a factory line model. It was realized that a "medicine nurse" could distribute drugs for a whole floor of patients with greater efficiency than could 10 nurses setting up separate medication trays for their patients.

The model had other specialist roles: the treatment nurse, the bedside caregiver, the temperature taker, the bed maker, and so forth. The theory was that a worker doing a limited number of tasks would grow expert at those tasks, improving the overall system efficiency. And the model achieved its goal: the greatest efficiency with the fewest workers. By dividing tasks, the model also allowed for creation of subordinate workers, those who might do the tasks requiring the least skill.

Eventually, several major flaws in the functional nursing system became evident—the most serious flaw was that the patient's needs did not fit into the role categories (medicines, treatments, baths) tended to fall through the cracks. In addition, patients suffered from personnel overload: too many people coming and going to perform too many different tasks. From the nurse's perspective, the problem with the factory model was that she never had a sense of a finished product. In essence, she felt like a factory worker.

It was not surprising when a new system eventually came into being. Predictably, it synthesized the best elements of private duty and functional nursing, eliminating the worst. *Team nursing* was created. In this system, nurses could have distinct products—patients of their own (somewhat like private duty). The whole patient would be served in his personhood, all his needs would be considered; he would no longer be a unit on an assembly line. And all this would occur because he would be exposed to fewer workers who knew him better: the team—his team.

Despite its attempt to correct the flaws of functional nursing, team nursing did not escape the task delegation design of functional nursing. True, it was the team leader, rather than the head nurse, who designated which team members would do which tasks; but that changed the leadership, not the focus on tasks delegation.

Yet in building a group, a team of members, each of whom knew "their patients" intimately, the system tried to superimpose the *patient focus* of private duty on the *task focus* of functional nursing. Still, the leadership decisions were focused on which team member should do what.

Because it is not a perfect world, the flaws of team nursing were bound to be discovered in time. Most of them related to the managerial and coordinating functions. Management had been pushed down the line from an experienced head nurse to a less-experienced team leader—a nurse not always comfortable delegating or managing people as a work team.

And, although fewer personnel saw every patient, the coordinating activities actually increased, because several people (registered nurse [RN] caregiver, nurse aide, RN team leader) might be involved with each patient without their roles and responsibilities being as clearly defined as in the old system. The team leader was eternally deciding anew who would do what. Coordination problems with other groups also increased, because team leaders tended to change from day to day, and physicians balked at never knowing with whom to discuss their patients' needs.

A few places tried to bandage the coordination problems with a miniature form of team nursing called *modular nursing*. Essentially, modular nursing carved out smaller teams—fewer nurses for fewer patients. This trend died quietly because it prevented flexible use of staff. Then, too, it offered nothing new because its structure was identical to that of team nursing.

It was inevitable that the next system of care assignment would be the antithesis of team. And so it was: *primary nursing* resolved the coordination and management problems of team nursing by a return to a patient-based, rather than task-based, work design. Namely, if a single nurse were responsible for a patient's care, then coordinating and assigning problems would be at a minimum.

Primary nursing (accompanied by an extensive thrust toward professional staffing) owed something to the health care environment of that time. Institutions were hiring more professional nurses, a feat made possible for several reasons. First, most insurance reimbursement systems paid costs incurred without questioning them. Second, nonprofessional staff, through active unionization, had received substantial salary increases. Suddenly the RN, who knew more, could do more, became cheap at the price. The argument for primary nursing went this way: If only one nurse were responsible for each patient and she was educationally prepared to complete all his care needs, then coordination needs fell away and patients got the best individualized care. In effect, we were back to private duty, the chief difference being that the primary nurse now had more than one patient.

The flaw in the primary nursing model became evident rather quickly: the primary nurse was present on the care unit for only about 40 out of 158 hours per week. The realities of the situation forced the primary nursing model to shift from a care *delivery* model to a care *planning* and *accountability* model. Actual care duties fell to others in the absence of the primary nurse, and sometimes even in her presence, if she had a heavy caseload.

TODAY'S PRACTICE ENVIRONMENT

We were about at that stage when today's nursing shortage (at first a shortage in available nurses, then a shortage in the number of nurses an institution could afford to hire) brought about a demand for change.

Restructured practice, not surprisingly, shows elements of all those systems that preceded it, and it synthesizes the preferred elements of team and primary care. What are the elements that have been adapted? First, restructured practice returns to the task orientation of team nursing. Indeed, that element is so strong it almost feels like a return to functional nursing. The principle is the same: division of tasks. But this time, the work division is more complex because the world of therapeutics, in the interim, has grown more specialized.

Despite its task orientation, restructured practice retains some of the patient focus of the primary system, often by keeping the planning and accountability function centered in a single nurse for each patient. Often she is the case manager. In this sense, the restructured practice models of today blend the two foci—the patient and the task. Figure 18–1 shows the rise and fall of historical assignment systems between the two parameters of a patient focus and a task focus.

It is useful to view the elements that drive our assignment systems through the theoretical model provided by Drucker (1974). He claimed that all work is designed around one of four motifs:

1. work and task
2. relations
3. results and performance
4. decisions (pp. 551–557).

Notice how Drucker's "design logics" (as he calls them) compare with Aristotle's (1958) formal, final, material, and efficient causes (pp. 31–34). Decisions start the process, that is, they are the efficient cause of management; work and task are the material causes; results and performance represent the final cause, whereas relations compose the formal cause. Although restructured practice rests solidly in the design logic of work and task, never before have we had a system that looks at all four of Drucker's design logics simultaneously in such a dramatic way.

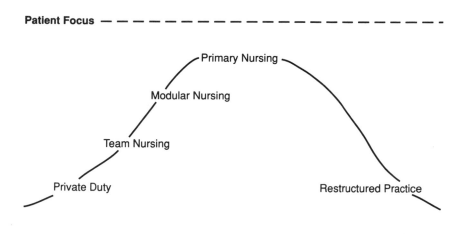

Figure 18–1. Care delivery models on dimensions of patient and task focus.

The system rests primarily in the design logic of *work and task* because, in all cases, the restructuring has involved a comprehensive look at what needs to be done, that is, the nitty-gritty tasks. Yet, more than in any prior system, what needs to be done is determined by the desired *results and performance.* (Hence, the introduction of case trajectory paths monitored by case managers with their eyes continuously on outcome goals.)

And—more than in any prior system—the question of who will do what (*relations*) is open for revision. There is intensive work concerning what *decisions* (and what sort of decisions) can be made by the various levels of worker, with a great downward shift in decision power occurring.

Although the balance is on the nuts and bolts, restructured practice is the closest we have ever come to a system balancing on several design logics simultaneously. Yet, make no mistake about it, the new system has more in common with functional nursing than with any other system. The commonalities are there. Both systems were designed to deal with an envisioned sustained shortage of professional nurses. Both focus on tasks, both have equally revolutionized the health care delivery of their respective eras.

REDESIGNING ROLES

Redesigning roles is the crux of the new system, with assignments made on the basis of the qualifications of the people who will do the tasks. The higher the preparation, the more complex the tasks.

The principle is one of safeguarding precious resources—in this case (as in functional nursing), the resource of professional nursing time.

Notice that in times when nurses earn comparatively low wages and there is no critical shortage of them, nurses are not treated as important resources. Because nurses tend to have a good work ethic and tend to be self-monitoring, it pays to use them as all-purpose workers. The trend of professional staffing pushed this strategy to the hilt. And it was successful—just as long as nurses were plentiful and their wages suppressed.

Then along came a shortage. Salaries increased, and it no longer made sense for employees to pay high hourly rates for personnel doing lower-level tasks. Enter once more neofunctional nursing (restructured practice).

We will look for a moment at some of the ways in which restructured nursing practice is being enacted. The modes are diverse, interesting, and even—some would say—exciting. One of the most interesting things is the way the pie is being sliced.

In the old functional system, every institution did it the same. Everyone had a medicine nurse, a treatment nurse, and so forth. In neofunctional nursing, each institution sees fit to make its own divisions of the pie. And the pies are being carved in all sorts of creative patterns. One of the things making for new arrangements in restructured practice is the *fact* of nursing specialty practice—not just for nurses holding master's degrees in specialties—but for all nurses.

There was a day when one could pull a general nurse from obstetrics and send her to a critical care unit. She might need a little guidance, but she would already have the essential skills. The same would be true for a nurse pulled from pediatrics to work in orthopedics. If a manager pulled a nurse to a different unit today, she would have a nurse who stared at new equipment, not knowing what to do with it. Specialism had occurred *de facto*.

What does specialism mean for restructured practice? It means that nurses are not as flexible as they once were. They cannot easily be moved from one unit to another. The flexible use of staff that used to be institution wide is now limited to a few similar units. Hence, restructured practice is no longer bound by the need to preserve flexibility of staff, an important criterion in its historical forerunner: functional nursing. But specialism is comfortable with restructured practice because the tasks of any given specialized nursing practice are different from the tasks of other specialized practices.

Let us look at restructured practice as it affects RN roles. The most limited sort of restructuring differentiates what 2-year and 3-

year nurses can do from what a 4-year nurse can do. This change is perhaps the least prevalent because it limits the use of some nurses. Nevertheless, it is occurring in many restructured practice plans. More typical is differentiated practice between an RN and a licensed practical nurse (LPN) or an RN and a nurse's aide.

Furthermore, institutions are creating new classifications of worker, called everything from patient care technician to environmental health worker. Many places, whether using RN-technician teams or RN–LPN teams, use a variant of Manthey's (1988) paired-partners concept.

Paired partners means that an RN has a permanent partner, LPN or nursing assistant, who invariably works with her. In other places, the partnership is between a senior baccalaureate-prepared nurse and a junior nurse (associate or diploma prepared). In places in which the luxury exists, the partner linkage is a function of the senior nurse's selecting her own partner member. In the idealized form of this practice, the permanent work team even shares the same duty schedule. Other places use the term *paired partners* more loosely, meaning two people who are assigned to work together on a given day.

In the more contained concept, the union is lasting and the RN is able to train the lower-level worker in what she wants done and how she wants it performed. In this way, tasks move to the lowest level, and tasks once seen as higher level can be done by lower-level personnel, if the number of such tasks is limited and the personnel are properly taught and supervised.

Another growing application of differentiated practice and paired partners involves a paired physician and RN. Sometimes this is called the *advanced practice model*. In the advanced practice model, the nurse member functions quite independently, with protocols negotiated and signed by her physician partner. The chief difference between this nurse and a primary nurse practitioner (when the partnered RN is not a practitioner) is that she functions in a primary and secondary mode—but only in conjunction with one physician. The partnership is not unlike the RN–LPN or RN–aide partnerships.

In the best of models, restructured practice extends beyond the nursing division, examining anew all the role functions of the institution. When new roles are carved, they may cross departmental lines previously not crossed. For example, a function once done by nurses may be shifted to laboratory workers, or erstwhile intern functions in the surgical suite may be shifted to an operating room technician. The broader the scope of roles considered, the more efficiency can be achieved by a reordering of tasks and roles.

Restructured practice is characterized by diversity, experimentation, decentralization to the lowest level, recognition of nursing specialism, and openness to the idiosyncrasies of both an institution and its practice environment.

STAFFING FACTORS

Let us look at staffing patterns, because they have undergone significant changes. The old system of primary care held out for professional staffing—decreasing use of auxiliary help so that each patient would be cared for by a professional nurse. The era featured general cutbacks of auxiliary help, not only in nursing but in other departments as well.

The greatest reorganization in restructured practice is occurring in skill mix reassessment, and the mix is typically shifting downward. Most of the new designing is done on an assumption that care needs will be provided by fewer professional nurses than in the old system. All design is aimed at preserving the limited resource of RNs—freeing them for direct care and essential decision making.

Primary nursing has had a longer life than professional staffing because it can be viewed as an accountability system instead of an assignment system. Actually, if the planning and evaluating elements are emphasized, then the primary nurse can delegate all sorts of actual care assignments to other personnel. In essence, the planning/evaluating model of primary nursing is compatible with any assignment system used in restructured practice.

As to roles for the RN, the greatest change is the newest role of case manager. This is a role that uses Drucker's (1974) design logic of performance and results, because it focuses directly on managing patient care outcomes.

SUMMARY

Restructured practice is the newest assignment system in acute care nursing. It is a reversion to a method with a task orientation. In general, nurses prefer the opposite pole of the continuum: the patient focus. When a shift is experienced toward the task orientation end of the polarity, it almost always indicates the press of environmental circumstances. And that has been the case today. The health care system is in the midst of adjusting its staffing mix. The answer to date has been that if nurses are paid more, they must expect to be fewer in number.

Because the restructured practice model involves more of Drucker's (1974) design logics than any previous model, the arrangements are complex, to say the least. The introduction of a case manager role (results-oriented model) has altered the management model from a hierarchical one to a matrix design. The head nurse (by whatever title) represents one authority line, whereas the case manager represents the other. The staff nurse is accountable to both authorities for her care.

Although matrix is an interesting managerial form, it always takes more maintenance work than does the hierarchical model. See, for example the descriptions of the complex relations involved in two such systems (Bunkers, 1992; Larson, 1992; Tonges, 1989a, 1989b).

Although restructured practice began in acute care, one can see elements of it spreading to long-term care delivery systems as they, too, cope with the same environmental stresses and scarcities.

Restructured practice, although not an ideal system, was probably as good a response to a difficult environment as could be made by the profession. That it is the most complex assignment system in our history is perhaps parallel to the fact that the rest of our health care industry is equally complicated.

REFERENCES

Aristotle (1958). Physics. In J. D. Kaplan (Ed.) & W. D. Ross (Trans.) *The Pocket Aristotle*. New York: Washington Square Press, a division of Simon and Schuster.

Bunkers, S. S. (1992). The healing web: A transformative model for nursing. *Nursing & Health Care, 2*, 68–73.

Drucker, P. F. (1974). *Management: Tasks, responsibilities, practices*. New York: Harper & Row.

Larson, J. (1992). The healing web—A transformative model: Part II. *Nursing & Health Care, 5*, 246–252.

Manthey, M. (1988). Primary practice partners: A nurse extender system. *Nursing Management, 3*, 58–59.

Tonges, M. C. (1989a). Redesigning hospital nursing practice: The professionally advanced care team (ProACT) model, Part 1. *Journal of Nursing Administration, 7*, 31–38.

Tonges, M. C. (1989b). Redesigning hospital nursing practice: The professionally advanced care team (ProACT) model, Part 2. *Journal of Nursing Administration, 9*, 19–22.

BIBLIOGRAPHY

Adams-Ender, C. L., Jennings, B., Bartz, C., & Jensen, R. (1991). Nursing practice models: The Army Nurse Corps experience. *Nursing & Health Care, 3*, 120–123.

American Academy of Nursing. (1991). *Differentiating nursing practice into the twenty-first century*. Kansas City, MO: Author.

Armstrong, D. M., & Stetler, C. B. (1991). Strategic considerations in developing a delivery model. *Nursing Economics, 2*, 112–115.

Curran, C. R. (1991). An interview with Karlene M. Kerfoot. *Nursing Economics, 3,* 141–147.

Johnson, M., Gardner, D., Kelly, K., Mass, M., & McCloskey, J. C. (1991). The Iowa model: A proposed model for nursing administration. *Nursing Economics, 4,* 255–262.

Newman, M. A., Lamb, G. S., & Michaels, C. (1991). Nurse case management: The coming together of theory and practice. *Nursing & Health Care, 8,* 404–408.

O'Malley, J., & Llorente, B. (1990). Back to the future: Redesigning the workplace. *Nursing Management, 10,* 46–48.

Sovie, M. D. (1990). Redesigning our future: Whose responsibility is it? *Nursing Economics, 1,* 21–26.

19 *Nursing Theory and Nursing Education*

Nursing education is presently undergoing a period of upheaval and change. We will look at two critical issues here: the changes in general nurse preparation and those in specialty education. Then we will leave the issue of trends and look at how theory may be used to structure and inform a curriculum and teaching methods.

CHANGES IN BASIC PREPARATION

The present change in basic student education mimics a polarity we have seen throughout this book. Indeed, it is similar to the competition between the nursing process and holistic theories—nursing process associated with taxonomies and quantitative measures, and holistic theories with qualitative measures and "softer" phenomena. The educational polarity is between the older, highly structured and science-based curricula and newer models often couched in New Age paradigms.

The dimensions of this polarity have been captured by Gould and Bevis (1992) and Munhall (1991) in similar terms, yet their conclusions are different. Gould and Bevis think the new paradigm will replace the old; Munhall, instead, has called for elbow room for everyone and being comfortable with our differences. The frames of reference of the two works are interesting, Munhall representing a school perspective, Gould and Bevis representing a state board decision. The two aspects are fitting, because change is happening on both fronts. Not only are faculty and state boards changing, but the leadership of the National League for Nursing (the accrediting body for schools of nursing) is also encouraging the new ideology.

*Barbara J. Stevens Barnum: NURSING THEORY:
ANALYSIS, APPLICATION, EVALUATION, FOURTH EDITION.*
© 1994, 1990, 1984, 1979 J.B. Lippincott.

Munhall has described the old ideology in terms such as measurement, behaviorism, Tylerism, pragmatism, the banking concept of information, and student submissiveness. She sees the new movement expressed in phenomenology, hermeneutics, feminist theory, caring philosophies, critical theory, symbolic interactionism, existentialism, and autonomous students. In brief, she has labeled the two ideologies as the behavioristic curriculum (older model) and the humanistic curriculum (newer model). For simplicity, I will use these two shorthand terms.

Gould and Bevis also have spoken of the behaviorist paradigm as favoring Tylerism, being objective driven, featuring hard-core behaviorism, detailing lists of all content items in curricula and classes, using lecture method, seeing the teacher as authority and practicing nurses as poor models, and deriving all learning from teacher-defined objectives. They have classified the new rules as involving less rigidity, learning goals instead of hard-line objectives, no rigid course outlines, a shift from evaluation to critique, participatory determination of appropriateness and progress among students and faculty, with curricula geared to critical thinking, creativity, meaning making, and caring.

Although the terms in these two articles are somewhat different, the discussions overlap. One might also track the polarity in Meyers, Stolte, Baker, Nishikawa, and Sohier (1991), who recommended a new curriculum based on learning strategies and thinking processes rather than content.

A related thorny issue, not usually addressed in the education literature, is the demand from practice executives that nurses be taught more of the high technology now used in acute care. Obviously, this demand is more in keeping with the older ideology and is unlikely to find much sympathy among advocates of the new one. In essence, these two factions (holding old and new ideologies) are struggling for position at the educational doors, and only time will tell the outcome. Will both groups learn to live together as Munhall suggests? Or will the New Age ideology overcome the older paradigm? At the moment, these seem the two most likely outcomes.

NURSE SPECIALIST EDUCATION

Another immediate issue on the educational plate concerns advanced practice and which role(s) will prevail: the clinical specialist model, the nurse practitioner pattern, or both. A brief look at the historical development these programs may be of use in clarifying the present status. For a detailed presentation of these differences, see Bullough (1992).

At their inception, clinical specialist programs focused on psychosocial needs. At the time, it seemed a great stride over the pathophysiologic perspective dominant in that era. Since that time, the role has become more well rounded, adding a strong scientific base to the original psychosocial aspects.

The practitioner movement, starting outside of nursing, has always had (as its nurse opponents are vocal in saying) a strong task orientation and a focus on pathophysiology. The added tasks have been those commonly performed by physicians. Nevertheless, bit by bit, most nurse practitioner programs have moved into mainstream nursing education, usually at the master's level. Because of this, students have had little chance to forget their nursing roots. And they, too, have been exposed to the psychosocial aspects of care.

In fact, the actual content of the clinical specialty programs and the related nurse practitioner programs (e.g., a pediatric clinical specialist program and a pediatric nurse practitioner program) have become more similar than dissimilar. When Forbes, Rafson, Spross, and Kozlowski (1990) compared nurse practitioner and clinical nurse specialist programs in gerontology and pediatrics, they found similar core requirements and minimal differences in content. As they noted, each curriculum had as its chief components the building of clinical judgment and leadership. Calkins (1984) also commented on the minor differences between the roles, with clinical nurse specialists prepared for more indirect client service, whereas nurse practitioners were prepared for more direct service.

Despite many educators being strongly committed to one or another of these roles, many schools are now converting to an advanced practitioner curriculum that contains the best of both programs and prepares the graduate for legal practitioner status. This joining of the two roles seems to be the trend of the future. The problem becomes one of developing one or more coherent nursing theories through which to enact the developing role. This is an instance in which the change in practice has outstripped and preceded the theoretical justification and conceptualization of the practice and the role.

Although these two issues seem to be those most contested in the educational marketplace, it is safe to say that there is great flux, even uncertainty, about just what directions will be set in education. Newer theories are making their mark on the scene, especially holistic, New Age, and feminist ideologies. It will be easier to judge the scene in a few years once the dust settles.

The rest of this chapter looks at the more traditional relationship between theory and education, beginning with their interface. Nursing theory and nursing education intersect in several ways. First, nursing theory (identified or assumed) is the subject matter of curriculum; second, in conjunction with educational theory, it organizes and designs the curricular plan. These two interfaces, respectively, determine the discipline model and the curriculum model of an educational program. In addition, nursing theory affects the teaching methods that are selected to convey information.

DISCIPLINE MODEL

Nursing theory is the subject matter of a nursing curriculum because it purports to teach nursing—for a certain level of practice, a specialized clinical area, or even a defined functional position. Whether faculty recognize it or not, a nursing curriculum conveys a theory (or theories) of nursing by virtue of the content selected.

The discipline model may be a specific nursing theory adopted (or adapted) from a given nurse theorist; it may be a model designed by the faculty; or it may be an intuited image of nursing. If an intuited image of nursing, the intuition may be shared among faculty, or individual faculty members may have differing images of nursing, bringing more than one discipline model into the curriculum.

The discipline model may be purposely brought to the foreground of the student's consciousness, or it may be unstated, assumed (perhaps not even clear to the faculty). When faculty members perceive nursing differently, the student may be exposed to different, even conflicting, images of nursing in different courses and clinical experiences within a single curriculum.

Consideration of a discipline model raises many questions: (1) Does the faculty need to be aware of the model(s) dominant in its teaching? Is it necessary for the student to recognize a model to learn its use? (2) Should the discipline model(s) be taught and made evident to the student? Or is a model adequately conveyed by the content selected under its auspices? (3) Should a single discipline model be selected for a given curriculum? Or should multiple models be allowed to coexist?

One or Many Discipline Models?

Having only one discipline model in a nursing program has several advantages. For one, it enables a faculty to better organize and select learning experiences. Furthermore, the model can serve as a criterion for evaluating student achievement. When a single model is the focus of group attention, its flaws are more likely to be corrected; it is more likely to be refined than when alternate models are used.

On the other hand, when each faculty member is allowed to select the nursing model of her choice, she may have more zest for teaching. Sophisticated students may enjoy seeing how diverse models function, whereas other students may be confused by the shifting images and approaches.

Obviously, a beginning student will have more difficulty adjusting to disparate models than will a more experienced student. Use of a single model enables the new student to integrate knowledge from diverse areas of study and facilitates her induction into the nursing milieu.

Use of a single model as the basis for a given first-level program does not preclude introducing the student to the fact that other nursing models exist. Indeed, it will help the student to understand the discipline model if she has other models with which to compare it. The other models, however, become informational content rather than models to be used in the student's practice. At the graduate level of nursing education, students should be sensitized to the effects of diverse models on nursing practice. Here, faculty have an obligation to make the student aware of multiple nursing models. Faculty may choose to do this by using two or more nursing models within the curriculum or, again, by using a single discipline model for the graduate program and introducing the student to other models as informational content.

In master's education, it is often the case that different study options in the same school will use different nursing models. For example, a psychiatric nursing program and a medical-surgical program are unlikely to select the same nursing model for advanced education. In such a setting, if students can freely elect courses outside of their own major, they can see different nursing models in action.

CURRICULUM MODEL

The curriculum model is the vehicle whereby the student is systematically introduced to the discipline model that dominates the program of study. The curriculum model distributes the content of a curriculum. An example follows.

Suppose that the faculty of a four-semester associate degree program elected to use Levine's (1971) theory of nursing as the discipline model in its program. Suppose, also, that for the curriculum model, Levine's four principles of conservation were selected, each as the basis for a single semester of study. In this case, the curriculum model and the discipline model would correspond.

An alternate approach would be one in which the content of the semesters was decided on a different principle (e.g., on the distribution of materials along a health–illness continuum) with Levine's principles (all four of them) being applied internally in each semester. Here, Levine's theory is still the discipline model, but the curriculum model no longer replicates the discipline model; it now contains another primary organizing principle—the health–illness continuum.

The curriculum model should facilitate learning of the discipline model if a single model has been selected. But that learning may or may not be improved when the curriculum model coincides with the discipline model. In the previous illustration, one might argue that the second curricular arrangement gives the student a better understanding of Levine's theory because all four conservation principles may be applied to every patient studied. In this instance, the curriculum model that differed from the discipline model better facilitated learning than did the direct application of the discipline model.

Often a curriculum model deviates from the discipline model to support learning theory. Also, some nursing theories simply are not formulated in a manner that provides for the distribution of curriculum elements. In these cases, the nursing theory will be subordinated to other organizing themes. The critical factor is that all organizing themes (primary and secondary) be compatible with each other.

Nursing Departments as the Basis of the Curriculum Model

When a faculty does not want to be limited to a single discipline model, a common practice is to use specialty departments as the primary organizing principles of the curriculum model. This produces a curriculum model with segments of the following sort: fundamentals of nursing, medical-surgical nursing, obstetrics, pediatrics, psychiatric nursing, and public health nursing. Suppose these blocks of study were used to organize a baccalaureate program, with the student moving from one segment to another sequentially, with little interplay among departments. What are the bases on which this curriculum model rests? The following theoretical designs might apply.

Area of Study	*Underlying Theory*
Fundamental of nursing	Skills (behavior-based)
Medical-surgical nursing	Body systems-based
Obstetric nursing	Life event-based
Pediatric nursing	Life phase-based
Psychiatric nursing	Patient behavior-based
Public health nursing	Epidemiology-based

With this curriculum model, every major block of study is derived from a different theoretical base. Such a curriculum presents nursing as a different subject in each course of study. Take, for example, the first two areas. In fundamentals, the students learn that nursing is the performance of skilled acts. Then in medical-surgical nursing, the primary divisions of study are determined by illnesses grouped according to body systems—respiratory disease, cardiovascular disease, and so forth. In many ways, the student is starting at step 1 again, finding out what nursing is.

For every block of study, the student's previous concepts of nursing will require revision; building on previous learning will be difficult. Each block of study will contain its own, unique programming for how one goes about nursing. The disadvantage of such an approach is that student learning may be slower; integration across course lines will not come easily. The advantage is that each block of study uses those theories that fit best with its subject matter.

Core Curriculum

When traditional departments are elected to form the curriculum model, attempts at unity often search for a *core* (shared notions or principles). It is presumed that this core can be taught first, unifying the diverse specialties. The argument usually fails in its application. Consider, for example, how the meaning of *stress* (a common core notion) changes when applied to the patient in labor, the community undergoing gentrification, the patient in anaphylactic shock, and the patient experiencing a life crisis. The instantiations are so different that prior generalized knowledge is meaningless; the applications are so unique that *stress* must be relearned in each instance. If the notion of core applies at all, it probably should be seen as a final synthesis rather than an initial generalization.

BUILDING A CURRICULUM MODEL

When the departmental structure is not used as the basis of the curriculum model, many alternatives may be used to organize an educational program. One source, the components of a discipline model, already has been mentioned. For example, one might organize an eight-component basic program around Johnson's (1980) behavioral subsystems: (1) affiliation, (2) aggression, (3) dependency, (4) achievement, (5) ingestion, (6) elimination, (7) sex, and (8) restoration. There are numerous schemes one could use to divide the curriculum pie:

1. skills and techniques
2. body systems or diseases

3. life events—developmental, crisis, other
4. life phases—birth to death
5. patient behaviors
6. locus of practice—environmental, institutional
7. steps of the nursing process—assessment, diagnosis, planning, intervention, evaluation
8. nursing goals—prevention, restoration, and sustenance

Other classifications may be imagined easily. Peplau (1965) identified 10 organizing themes for curricula that still hold today:

1. area of practice
2. organs and bodily systems
3. age of client
4. degrees of illness
5. length of illness
6. nurse activities
7. fields of knowledge
8. subroles of the work role of the staff nurse
9. professional goals
10. clinical services

Few curricula are organized along a single dimension. More often, two or three organizing themes are crosshatched to build a curriculum grid. Table 19–1 illustrates a curriculum in which selected patient problems form primary organizing threads.

A second organizing principle has been woven through the selected problems; in this case, life phases. In this curriculum, courses might be organized around patient problems, or reversed and organized around life phases. In Table 19–2, another curriculum model interweaves the organizing themes of the traditional body systems and the nursing process. Not all themes are compatible with each other. It is impossible, for example, to have two contradictory processes (e.g., nursing process *and* problem solving) in a single model.

Every nursing education program should be able to identify the discipline model(s) and curriculum model that underlie the content of the program. When uniformity is sought in a curriculum, these structural aspects provide the matrix for it. When diversity is allowed or even encouraged, it is even more important that students recognize the different ideologies and shifts in the meaning of nursing.

CURRICULUM SEQUENCING

Whatever discipline model a faculty wishes to convey to the student body, it must do so in a manner that is educationally sound. Hence,

Table 19-1. Curriculum Model Cross-Gridding Patient Problems and Life Phases.

| | Dominant Threads: Patient Problems | | | | |
Secondary threads: Life phases	Problems of oxygenation and nutrition	Problems related to activities of daily living and mobility	Problems of fluid balance and elimination	Problems of self-image and role fulfillment	Problems of pain and discomfort
Infancy					
Childhood					
Adolescence					
Adulthood					
Senior citizen status					

Table 19-2. Curriculum Model Cross-Gridding Body Systems and Nursing Process.

Dominant Threads: Body Systems

Secondary threads: steps of the nursing process	Skeletal system	Integumentary system	Circulatory system	Respiratory system	Alimentary system	Excretory system	Endocrine/ reproductive system
Nursing assessment							
Nursing diagnosis							
Nursing care planning							
Nursing intervention							
Nursing evaluation							

an interplay necessarily occurs between theory of nursing and theory of education.

A major design problem in a basic nursing curriculum model is the selection of the entry point and sequencing of content. It is difficult to introduce the novice to nursing because the practice setting is rich in complexity and cannot be artificially simplified for the benefit of the learner. Even a "simple" patient interacts with a complex, unpredictable, and multidimensional environment. Because nursing situations are inherently rich and complex, it is difficult to know where to start.

Curriculum organization attempts to give order and sequence in a way that is meaningful to the novice learner. Nursing is more than simply new knowledge content for a beginning student; it is a new milieu, a new role, a new world.

Perhaps the very complexity of nursing phenomena accounts for the stress that nursing educators place on the need for moving from *simple to complex* in organizing nursing curricula. Like many self-evident rules, the dictate to move from simple to complex is easier to prescribe than to follow. The use of such an educational prescription has impact on content sequencing.

Suppose a program attempts to move from simple to complex by starting with a study of the cell; progressing to tissues (groups of cells); then to organs (groups of tissues); then to integrated systems (groups of organs); and finally, to the totally functional man (groups of integrated systems). The notion of simple to complex considered here starts with simple building bricks (cells) and works toward the more complex entities.

Consider, however, what happens to the nursing content with this design. The student would be likely to study hemolytic diseases and renal failures early in the program (cellular phenomena); heart failure later (organ impairment); and fractures of the extremities (integrated systems of the body) much later.

The intended logic of simple to complex is confounded here, because the hemolytic and renal cellular diseases are more complex than is heart failure (a mechanical problem), and the mechanics of heart failure are more complex than is the simple fracture (integrated systems of bone and muscle providing mobility). In addition, movement from cellular to integrated systems contradicts another educational dictate—moving from the known to the unknown. Suppose, now, that the simple-to-complex dictate were to be applied in a curriculum with a life-phase focus. In this curriculum, the study of the ill child clearly should occur *later* than study of the ill adult, because illness in a growing and developing organism is more complex. In this case, however, logical age sequence would dictate a different order: movement from birth to senescence. Again, the simple-to-complex dictate contradicts another principle, in this case, the notion of logical sequence.

Another curriculum might move from wellness to progressively serious illness in an attempt to traverse from simple to complex. Yet one is reminded of Freud, who studied psychology in the ill rather than the well, because the maladies were more plainly evident in the extreme cases. Hence, applying the dictate of simple to complex in moving from health to illness contradicts the educational principle of moving from the obvious to the more subtle. The self-evident needs of the ill may be simpler for the novice nurse to recognize and understand than are the more subtle health needs of the well.

The application of educational prescriptions in nursing curricula is not so simple as one might wish. In all three illustrations, a single educational prescription (simple to complex) contradicted other principles. The same would be true had we taken another principle as illustration.

LEARNING REQUIREMENTS

Because nursing is a practice profession, nursing education is necessarily education for action. What is learned in nursing can be grossly divided into three categories: (1) cognitive content, (2) psychomotor tasks, and (3) judicious application of both in the extant nursing setting. Here, *cognitive content* refers to all that information the nurse learns as background to her functioning (e.g., anatomy, physiology, pathology, psychology, medical procedures, nursing techniques, and patient diagnoses). It is the knowledge she learns, not for its own sake, but so that she will have enough information with which to make accurate clinical judgments later. *Psychomotor tasks* include those specific learned acts that nurses perform according to a given rationale by applying accepted techniques (e.g., administering medications and treatments, implementing diagnostic procedures). These acts are primarily mechanical. The third sort of learning, *judicious application* of cognitive knowledge and psychomotor skills in extant settings, is more complex than the other two kinds of learning. This sort of learning clearly is the seat of independent nursing practice. It also represents the sort of knowledge that is most difficult to acquire and teach. The learning skills required here are recognizing, interpreting, and adapting. Three instances of these nursing skills are examined here: (1) red flagging, (2) labeling, and (3) responding.

Red Flagging

Red flagging refers to the recognition that a problem situation exists. An instance of its absence may serve to illustrate it. I once observed a nurse diligently complete a nursing history for a patient, during which she asked if the patient had any chronic health problems. The patient responded negatively. Two questions later, she asked if he were routinely taking any medications. The patient said that he took Aldactazide daily. The nurse wrote in this fact and continued down the form. No red flag was raised in her mind when a patient who claimed *no* chronic health problem admitted to taking a drug daily. This nursing failure cannot be accounted for simply as a lack of knowledge concerning the drug. Whether or not she knew the drug, she should have recognized the inconsistency in the patient's two responses.

Labeling

Labeling occurs when a nurse interprets a concrete situation by virtue of previously acquired concepts. Again, acquisition of the pertinent concept(s) does not ensure application in the clinical setting. For example, the nurse may have a general conception of *denial*, but something specific in the patient's behavior must trigger the nurse's judgment that a case of denial actually exists. This form of nursing activity (interpreting) is complex in that knowledge and understanding of a concept is not the nursing activity; instead, identification of the cognitive concept in its unique instantiation is the desired outcome.

Nursing knowledge consists of recognizing the diverse and varying instances in terms of the concept. Psychic states such as denial, anxiety, and euphoria take different forms in different patients. Similarly, physiologic states vary in symptomatology from patient to patient. The teacher must understand that a student cannot be assumed to have learned a concept merely because she was able to identify a single (or even several) instantiations.

Responding

Recognizing (red flagging) and interpreting (labeling) nursing phenomena are only two aspects of successful independent nursing practice. *Responding* is a third important measure. An illustration follows. I once observed the behaviors of a nursing staff caring for a patient on absolute voice rest. Each nurse who entered the room reminded the patient of the need for voice rest—often after she had posed questions that required verbal responses. Hence, the nurses' own behaviors elicited the forbidden response, triggering their subsequent reminders to the patient. Only one nurse developed a successful response pattern to the situation. She used the technique of whispering to the patient, the deviation in her own vocal behavior serving as a constant and successful reminder to the patient.

Red flagging, labeling, and responding form a bridge between cognitive content (abstract and general) and extant instantiations of that content (concrete and specific). Because the essence of nursing is in its application, nursing education should focus on building clinical skills such as these.

TEACHING STRATEGIES

What teaching strategies are necessary to convey the required learning in nursing? The answers are simple for cognitive content and psychomotor skills. Cognitive content is easily transmitted through a variety of media: lectures, discussions, programmed learning, or reading assignments. For the average student, acquisition of cognitive content can be achieved in the absence of skilled teaching, provided an alternative information source, such as a good text, is available. Psychomotor skills, on the other hand, require demonstration, return demonstration with corrective feedback, and skill development through practice. Few psychomotor skills of nursing are difficult, although some, such as scrubbing in the operating room, require the learning of intricate, stylized behaviors.

Learning to apply cognitive knowledge and psychomotor skills judiciously in the extant nursing setting, however, is a different matter. This is a complex learning task in which the nurse improves over time, learning from each clinical instance in which recognizing (red flagging), interpreting (labeling), or adapting (responding) occurs. The major teaching effort in nursing should occur in the clinical setting. Cases can be selected to allow the student to practice these skills. The actual clinical case is preferable to written or audiovisual case studies.

Yet not every case study uses an actual patient. And contrived case studies (simulations or written cases) may or may not actually teach clinical behaviors, depending on their structures. Some instructors use nursing cases merely as devices to transmit normative, cognitive content. This happens when a typical patient is selected, and teaching the care of this patient follows the average pattern in all respects. Such a case study is really a lecture in disguise.

In a real case study, the uniqueness and variations presented by a patient are the important factors. To teach the skills of recognizing, interpreting, and adapting, the important factor is not that the patient has a particular condition or problem, but that the case as presented is inconsistent, incomplete, miscast, or inadequately managed to achieve goals. The idiosyncrasies of the clinical patient inevitably intrude on a good study. Cases can be created that test important clinical thinking skills, but they take a lot of planning.

It is helpful if the thought process behind the teaching–learning strategy and the thought process used in nursing practice coincide. That way, the student can practice those thought patterns as she learns. A teaching strategy that uses one thought pattern cannot teach a student to use a different pattern. For example, a didactic lecture on the steps of problem solving will not teach the student to problem solve. Indeed, the teacher's behavior identifies no problem, uses no solution-seeking procedures, and does not present the subject matter as problematic. We will examine briefly some teaching strategies that exemplify dialectic, logistic, problematic, and operational thought patterns.

The appropriate thought pattern for students to learn in any given curriculum is dictated by the nature of the accepted discipline model, in other words, the nursing theory used in the curriculum. In the classroom, correspondence will not occur unless it is planned. But if it is planned, the learning experience serves a dual function—teaching content and process simultaneously.

Some teaching strategies are flexible enough to express more than one method. Lecture, for example, can be made to express any given thought mode simply by controlling the organization and plan of presentation. But some strategies are naturally good fits with specific methods of thought.

A Dialectic Teaching Strategy

The traditional dialectic teaching strategy is the dialogue or Socratic method. In dialogue, the teacher leads the student to develop and expand her own thoughts on a given subject, primarily by the use of well-constructed questions and demonstrations of inconsistencies in, or contradictions to, the student's position. Dialogue proceeds through self-revelation, the student's insight being prodded by the teacher's use of added perspectives or challenges. In dialogue, the student moves from a narrow conception of her subject matter to broader and more comprehensive understandings that encompass more events and more complexities.

Contrary to popular use of the term, dialogue is not simply any conversational interchange; it is an interchange that assimilates new information into a synthesis with previous knowledge. Such synthesis is not merely additive in nature, because the previously held knowledge is itself altered by the new information.

Logistic Teaching Strategies

A curriculum using the concept of mastery learning is logistic in design. This teaching strategy divides the components to be learned into an invariant learning sequence in which acquisition of Component A is a necessary prerequisite to acquisition of Component B, hence using the systems-building technique.

Another logistic educational strategy is the use of programmed instruction. Linear programs feed the student clearly defined components of the knowledge system, one at a time, providing for reinforcement and testing of each component as the program progresses. As components are added and related to each other, the total knowledge system is amassed.

Most computer-assisted instruction programs, and some interactive audiovisual programs, follow a similar logistic system of assembling building blocks. When branching logic is used, one can see the influence of an operational system instead.

Formative testing is a logistic teaching strategy in which the course is conceived of as consisting of separate and definite units. Tests are constructed to measure attainment for each given unit. Individually prescribed instruction is offered for those units in which the student fails to show the required mastery.

All logistic teaching strategies demonstrate a concern with individual units and their interrelationships. Elaborate systems may be constructed from the given components, but the focus is on learning the components and their relationships.

Problematic Teaching Strategies

A problematic teaching strategy involves the student actively in solving problems. The most common strategy is the use of the case study. The case study usually focuses on the circumstances of a single patient, the objective being to resolve that situation into one in which the patient has all his problems solved. The case study may be used in a single class or it may dominate the whole curriculum.

The case study—more properly, the problem study—is a strategy that allows extensive manipulation on the part the teacher. For beginning students, she may identify the problems, letting the students seek solutions. Or she may use the case as a problem-seeking exercise, teaching students how to find the important factors among the array of available data.

Another means of variation in the problem study has to do not with the presence or absence of components, but with the form in which the components arise. For example, presentation of the problem can vary on a continuum from a clear statement of the problem as given, or problem containment in a simple situation, to problem containment in a complex situation. Additionally, the problem itself may vary in complexity.

Mind-set also affects the level of difficulty of the problem. For example, if a student knows that a given case is being used in the study of defense mechanisms, she is likely to locate and define the defense mechanism with greater ease than she would in a case assigned to her in a different context.

The problem study also varies depending on whether it occurs in a natural or an attenuated environment. No written problem study displays an environment as complex as an actual patient case. Simulated patients come closer, but even they are scripted with limited information. The student also might be given a real problem to work out in actual clinical case.

The teacher can encourage problematic thought by the design of her classroom lectures. Lecture material can be presented in the problematic mode, stating a problem and working through the steps to its solution. This gives students an opportunity to observe someone else using the problematic mode. Demonstrations also can be given, not as step-by-step procedures, but as the presentation of an objective and determination of various appropriate ways to reach that objective.

Operational Teaching Strategies

The operational mode focuses on the perspective of the agent. Debate typifies this mode by presenting opposing perspectives on the same topic. Similarly, a symposium uses speakers with different, although not necessarily opposing, perspectives on the same subject matter.

Other operational forms focus on differences in the activities of the learner. Teaching by educational games is an example of competitive activities. Such games are used in teaching nurse managers (although they are seldom adapted to clinical education). They involve actual moves and countermoves by opposing learners. The objective, as in the debate, is to beat the opponent. Some educational games are played with human opponents; others have computerized opponents in the form of a program of moves and countermoves.

The in-basket exercise is a noncompetitive operational strategy used in the teaching of nurse managers. It may be contrasted with the problematic mode in the following way. Although the in-basket exercise may require problem-solving activity, the focus is not on a single problem and its definition and resolution. Instead, the focus is on a constellation of activities that may include solving problems as well as other actions, such as processing multiple pieces of information and selecting some items for attention but eliminating others. What is evaluated is not simply the adequacy of the solution of one or more selected problems, but the total performance—the whole sequence of varied activities on the part of the participant.

SUMMARY

Nursing theory and nursing education intersect in many dimensions. Only a few have been addressed in this chapter. The movement to free up curricula from some of the stringent conditions required in the past does not break this relationship, although it may call for different decisions concerning theory. An informed curriculum with thoughtful interface with theory and other curricular elements provides a coherent approach to educational design.

REFERENCES

Bullough, B. (1992). Alternative models for specialty nursing practice. *Nursing & Health Care, 5,* 254–259.

Calkins, J. D. (1984). A model for advanced nursing practice. *Journal of Nurse Administration, 1,* 24–30.

Forbes, K. E., Rafson, J., Spross, J. A., & Kozlowski, D. (1990). Clinical nurse specialist and nurse practitioner core curricula survey results. *Nurse Practitioner, 4,* 43–48.

Gould, J. E., & Bevis, E. O. (1992). Here there be dragons. *Nursing & Health Care, 3,* 126–133.

Levine, M. E. (1971). Holistic nursing. *Nursing Clinics of North America, 2,* 253–264.

Meyers, S. T., Stolte, K. M., Baker, C., Nishikawa, H., & Sohier, R. (1991). A process-driven curriculum in nursing education. *Nursing & Health Care, 9,* 460–463.

Munhall, P. (1991, January). *A new age ism: Beyond a toxic apple.* Paper presented at the faculty development conference, Orlando, FL.

Johnson, D. E. (1980). The behavioral system model for nursing. In J. P. Riehl & C. Roy (Eds.), *Conceptual models for nursing practice* (2nd ed., pp. 207–216). New York: Appleton-Century-Crofts.

Peplau, H. (1965). Specialization in professional nursing. *Nursing Science, 4,* 268–187.

20 Theory, Research, and Knowledge

Theory, research, and knowledge are intricately related phenomena. How one acquires knowledge (*epistemology*) is influenced by one's notion of reality (*ontology*). And the sort of research recognized as valid in reaching conclusions determines the type of theory a nurse will select. There is little agreement about what methods produce warranted knowledge or about what reality is like. Hence, it is easy to account for the plethora of nursing theories. Let us start with a quick look at ontology to see where the disagreements originate.

REALISM VERSUS CONCEPTUALISM

Generally, two opposing ontologies appear in the literature on nursing theory: realism and conceptualism. The two approaches are different and irreconcilable. In realism, one believes that the world exists "out there," independent of the knower. Research and theory seek to discover and explain the nature of that external reality.

In conceptualism, reality does not exist independent of the knower. Invention, rather than discovery, is the dominant mode of knowing reality. The two concepts are the extreme poles, with all sorts of variations on the continuum that spans them. Any ontology affects the kinds of nursing theories adopted and the methods selected for research.

Calling them *scientific paradigms*, Newman (1992) separated out three ontologic positions that have particular pertinence to nursing. The first is the *particulate-deterministic* view, describing phenomena as "isolatable, reducible entities having definable properties that can be measured." (p. 10) Newman's intermediate position, the *inter-*

Barbara J. Stevens Barnum: NURSING THEORY:
ANALYSIS, APPLICATION, EVALUATION, FOURTH EDITION.
© 1994, 1990, 1984, 1979 J.B. Lippincott.

active-integrative paradigm, "views reality as multidimensional and contextual. It acknowledges the importance of experience and includes both subjective and objective phenomena." (p. 11) In her third category, the *unitary-transformative*, "the human being is viewed as unitary and evolving as a self-organizing field, embedded in a larger self-organizing field. . . . Knowledge is personal. . . . Inner reality depicts the reality of the whole." (p. 11) To isolate these three spots on the continuum is particularly useful in nursing, because they mark the basic world views under which most nursing theories can be classified.

RESEARCH AND THE NATURE OF REALITY

The diverse ontologic positions described all have their own methods for validating knowledge. Popper (1953), a philosopher who falls into the camp of the realists (or under Newman's particulate-deterministic paradigm), made the following link between a reality that is "out there" and the method of knowing it. Because all of reality is objective, Popper has asserted, all research involves the same process. He therefore holds social scientists to the same methodology as bench scientists (i.e., to repeatable experiments to be confirmed or refuted by controlled experiments):

> The only course open to the social sciences is to forget all about the verbal fireworks and to tackle the practical problems of our time with the help of the theoretical methods which are fundamentally the same in all sciences. I mean the methods of trial and error, of inventing hypotheses which can be practically tested, and of submitting them to practical tests. A social technology is needed whose results can be tested by piecemeal social engineering (p. 365).

Popper's philosophy of realism sees the world as given:

> Scientific results are "relative" . . . only in so far as they are the results of a certain stage of scientific development and liable to be superseded in the course of scientific progress. But this does not mean that truth is "relative." If an assertion is true, it is true forever (p. 364).

Dewey's (1938) reality and his method (problematic) differ from Popper's. For Dewey, the result has precedent over method:

> We are able to contrast various kinds of inquiry that are in use or that have been used in respect to their economy and efficiency in reaching warranted conclusions. We know that some methods of inquiry are better than others in just the same way in which we know that some methods of surgery, farming, road-making, navigating or what-not are better than others. It does not follow in any of these cases that the "better" methods are ideally perfect, or that they are regulative or "nor-

mative" because of conformity to some absolute form. They are the methods which experience up to the present time shows to be the best methods available for achieving certain results (p. 104).

For Dewey, inquiry is

the controlled or directed transformation of an indeterminate situation into one that is so determinate in its constituent distinctions and relations as to convert the elements of the original situation into a unified whole (pp. 104–105).

This process occurs through an interaction between ideas and facts. (This would place Dewey in Newman's middle range, interactive-integrative paradigm.)

Some observed facts point to an idea that stands for a possible solution. This idea evokes more observations. Some of the newly observed facts link up with those previously observed and are such as to rule out other observed things with respect to their evidential function. The new order of facts suggests a modified idea (or hypothesis) which occasions new observations whose results again determines [sic] a new order of facts, and so on until the existing order is both unified and complete (Dewey, 1938, p. 113).

Although Popper's scientific method seeks to find out about a reality separate from his inquiry into it, Dewey's reality is itself changed in the process of inquiry. Method and reality are not separate:

The transformation is existential and hence temporal. The precognitive unsettled situation can be settled only by modification of its constituents. Experimental operations change existing conditions. . . . Only execution of existential operations directed by an idea in which ratiocination terminates can bring about the re-ordering of environing conditions required to produce a settled and unified situation. . . .

    . . . knowledge is related to inquiry as a product to the operations by which it is produced (Dewey, 1938, p. 118).

For Dewey, the inquiry itself produces the reality; it is not something "out there," totally separate from the investigation. Reality is an interaction between inquirer and environment. Bergson (1955), another philosopher, has presented a third view of reality and methods of inquiry:

Philosophers, in spite of their apparent divergencies, agree in distinguishing two profoundly different ways of knowing a thing. The first implies that we move round the object; the second that we enter into it. The first depends on the point of view at which we are placed and on the symbols by which we express ourselves. The second neither depends on a point of view nor relies on any symbol. The first kind of knowledge may be said to stop at the relative; the second, in those cases where it is possible, to attain the absolute (p. 21).

Bergson (1955) has illustrated what is meant by absolute knowledge:

> Were all the translations of a poem into all possible languages to add together their various shades of meaning and, correcting each other by a kind of mutual retouching, to give a more and more faithful image of the poem they translate, they would yet never succeed in rendering the inner meaning of the original (pp. 22–23).

Bergson refers to intuitive knowing as intellectual sympathy. Obviously, this method of knowing is far different from the methods previously examined:

> If there exists any means of possessing a reality absolutely instead of looking at it from outside points of view, of having the intuition instead of making the analysis; in short, of seizing it without any expression, translation, or symbolic representation—metaphysics is that means. Metaphysics, then, is the science which claims to dispense with symbols (Bergson, 1955, p. 24).

Bergson's reality is different from either Popper's or Dewey's:

> This reality is mobility. Not things made, but things in the making, not self-maintaining states, but only changing states, exist. Rest is never more than apparent, or, rather, relative. The consciousness we have of our own self in its continual flux introduces us to the interior of a reality, on the model of which we must represent other realities. All reality, therefore, is tendency, if we agree to mean by tendency an incipient change of direction (pp. 49–50).

Bergson's world is at the far end of the pole in conceptualism, reminding us of Newman's unitary-transformative world view. Here, then, are three different world views and three different views of how inquiry rightly occurs. In each case, the acceptable method of research depends on the sort of reality assumed. The conception of reality dictates the nature of methods perceived as appropriate for the acquisition of knowledge.

THEORY AND RESEARCH

Theory and research form a recycling chain in which theory directs research, research corrects theory, and corrected (or confirmed) theory directs more research. But a theory cannot be subjected to direct testing. Instead, one reasons that if Theory X is true, then Consequences Q, R, and S will follow under Conditions A and B. One then tests through research to see if these predicted consequences actually occur under Conditions A and B. If the consequences predicted by the theory hold up under rigorous research conditions, then the theory is confirmed.

Of course, someone else may always come along later with an equally logical (or better) explanation of why Consequences Q, R, and S occurred under Conditions A and B. Theories are not proven; they are confirmed. Confirmation (or validation) simply means that, no cases to the contrary, a theory is accepted as an explanation of a phenomenon until a better explanation comes along. Seekers after eternal truth had better not rely on the research-theory cycle.

What are the outcomes of research? One possible outcome is that an original theory may be disproved or require modification as a result. Often the researcher is not so fortunate to recognize why a theory did not work or how it must be modified. Nevertheless, a theory disproved is a positive research outcome because it eliminates one false lead.

On the other hand, in finding one theory invalid, a researcher may formulate an entirely new theory as she gains insight into the relationships among the variables under study. The new theory may itself suggest further nursing research. Any given research may confirm a theory, disprove a theory, suggest modifications to a theory, or suggest development of an entirely new theory.

All theories are not testable. Some may arise with a subject matter and method that make the testing formidable. Think, for example, of the medievalists who tried to find irrefutable proof for the existence of God. For other theories, the research that would constitute confirmation may be imagined, but impossible. The research Einstein conceptualized to support his theories was not possible until decades later, when appropriate measuring devices had been invented.

NURSING: TWO CAMPS

In nursing, there has been a tendency to divide theories and research into two camps, the one close to the positivist (realist) view, the other close to the conceptualist view. Each "side" has developed its own theory base using different techniques in seeking knowledge.

The positivist view is driven by the classical experimental design, hypothesis testing, and what gets termed *the scientific method*—hard science, in other words—with controls, quantitative procedures, and statistical manipulations. There are variations on the experimental design, of course, because there are situations in which variables simply cannot be manipulated. Retrospective analysis of data is one way around the problem. Whatever its design, the quantitative method looks at the component parts of the phenomena under study, seeking to describe the interrelationships among them. The objective is to create explanatory theory and, where possible, situation-producing theory.

For much of our history, nurse researchers at this pole (labeled as positivism, empiricism, or quantitative research) opposed what they perceived as soft science and soft methods, in other words, subject matter that was not strictly objective and methods that were not quantitative. Eventually nursing reached a compromise position in which both sorts of research and both world views were accepted as valid pursuits by the majority of nurses. The quantitative versus qualitative debate became an issue of preferences instead of right versus wrong. Now, ironically, some researchers on the qualitative end are trying to suppress quantitative research in nursing.

Qualitative studies (focused on subject matter conceived closer to the conceptualist end of the continuum) started off with phenomenalism as the chief method of inquiry. So-called grounded research (becoming immersed in the phenomena under study) grew in popularity. That popularity continues today, but, by now, we have at least two new versions of phenomenology, each with its own particular twist. To understand how hermeneutics and critical theory differ from each other and from phenomenology, we look first at the original system.

PHENOMENOLOGY

Phenomenology, a method of inquiry frequently associated with existential and holistic theories, sees the inquirer's direct experience of a thing as a legitimate way of coming to know it. It is an epistemology as well as a method of research. It asserts that things must be known in their entirety rather than by reduction to their parts.

Phenomenology reinstates the primacy of the subjective qualities of the matter under consideration. It is a deliberate effort to set aside scientific interpretations that reduce an entity to component parts; it preserves the view of the subject matter as experienced by the inquirer.

Phenomenology maintains that experience and the thing to which it refers are inseparably linked. It is concerned with the phenomenon experienced rather than its referent. Focus is not on the thing-in-itself, but on the thing-as-experienced (Kant, 1953, pp. 78–89). Cohen (1987) has added that "this is not mystical but involves logical insight based on careful consideration of representative examples." (p. 31) Phenomenology may be applied to an object or an abstraction. One can explore a meteorite or abstract concepts such as beauty or human anxiety. Phenomenology seeks to reveal a thing in all its dimensions, in all its richness.

Paterson and Zderad (1976) were early advocates of the phenomenologic method, which they called *humanistic* nursing. More recently, Benner (1985) stated the limitation of the positivist view:

> The paradox of the subject/object split of Cartesian dualism is that it is either extremely subjectivizing or extremely objectifying. The self is viewed as a possession and attributes are given objectively as possessions by the subject in a purely intentional way. This view cannot take account of the historical, cultural, embodied, situated person (p. 2).

HERMENEUTICS

Hermeneutics is a derivation of phenomenology that is popular among nurse theorists. In essence, hermeneutics interprets human phenomena not to uncover universal laws, but to explicate context, producing understanding rather than knowledge of the subject under enquiry. Hermeneutics aims to produce understanding through agreed-on interpretation of the meaning of events taken in context. Rabinow and Sullivan (1987) have described the movement this way:

> For the human sciences both the object of investigation—the web of language, symbol, and institutions that constitutes signification—and the tools by which investigation is carried out share inescapably in the same pervasive context that is the human world (p. 6).

And interpretations begin

> from the postulate that the web of meaning constitutes human existence to such an extent that it cannot ever be meaningfully reduced to constitutively prior speech acts, dyadic relations, or any other predefined elements (Rabinow & Sullivan, 1987, p. 6).

Rabinow and Sullivan see meaning as laying somewhere between the subjective minds of the actors and "out there." As they have said, "These meanings are intersubjective; they are not reducible to individual subjective psychological states, beliefs, or propositions. They are neither subjective nor objective but what lies behind both." (p. 7) They have characterized hermeneutics as a system that can:

> heighten the contrast between knowledge seen as technical project. . . and knowledge seen, in the human sciences, as inescapably practical and historically situated (p. 2).
>
> Holistic explanation in the new forms seek to organize a wide variety of human phenomena that cannot be comprehended through models based on linear relations among elements (p. 5).

Patterson (1991) has offered the following three criticisms of hermeneutics:

1. Criteria for judgment of interpretations are lacking.
2. There are political objections to interpretive social science.
3. It fails the criterion for empirical social science.

CRITICAL SOCIAL THEORY

The next derivative method arising out of phenomenology and hermeneutics is called *critical theory* or *critical social theory*. The goal of this method is to free the knower from the influences of societal ideologies that may have biased his or her thinking. Often this variant is advocated in feminist theories that envision distortions arising from the false overlay of values and behaviors in a patriarchal society.

Although the notion of correcting distortions in perception is wise, one must understand that some theorists use the method to justify their own agendas of advancing feminism. The researcher may be invited to exchange one interpretive lens for another. In essence, critical theory has a worthy goal, but that goal may be undermined if the researcher is invited to correct for distortions of one ideology only to substitute another ideology in its place.

RECAPITULATION

In general, then, these qualitative positions on research contrast with the methods clustering around the realism polarity. Kim (1990) defined the field of nursing research as cast on three philosophical paradigms: analytical empiricism, Heideggerian phenomenology, and critical social theory (p. 2). These three points are not a bad summary of the most popular positions today.

Ironically, we have completed a circle in nursing, with qualitative research and related holistic theories replacing quantitative approaches in popularity. One reason that quantitative positions are "at risk" is that, for a long time, their strongest advocates followed a narrow form of logical positivism—long since moribund in philosophy where it arose.

Jacox (1974) was an early advocate of logical positivism (or the *Received View* as it came to be known). This form of positivism was a rather simplistic, building-blocks, logistic formulation. Jacox, at that time, identified these three rules of theory construction:

1. Specify, define, and classify the concepts used in describing the phenomena of the field.
2. Develop statements or propositions that propose how two or more concepts are related.

3. Specify how all of the propositions are related to each other in a systematic way (p. 5).

This model continued to be dominant in nursing for many years. In 1978, for example, Fawcett wrote,

> A theory is defined as "a set of interrelated (concepts), definitions, and propositions that present a systematic view of phenomena by specifying relations among variables." An empirically tested theory is composed of concepts that are narrowly bounded, specific and explicitly interrelated (p. 50).

None of this is to say that the logistic, building-blocks method of theory development is wrong; it is simply to say that the logistic system of thinking is only one way among many to formulate theory. Even Jacox (Webster, Jacox, & Baldwin, 1984) admitted this in a criticism of the received view):

> In retrospect it can be seen that several basic assumptions underlying the tenets of the Received View are traceable to the seventeenth-century world view. These assumptions were so basic to Received View practice that they were seldom explicitly articulated; they are the presuppositions of Received View doctrines.
>   Among these assumptions is the seventeenth-century emphasis on independence and atomicity, or the primacy of parts in comparison with the wholes which can be formed with them. Another is that mathematics is the language of nature. From this belief the tenet that theories ought to be formalized is a direct sequence (p. 28).

Overreliance on the logistic formulation of theories in nursing served to denigrate theories that were not logistic in form. Or worse, it caused theorists or their advocates to reinterpret their theories in a logistic format, causing distortions in otherwise interesting theories. The problem was that the holders of this perspective tried to sell it as the only right way. Nurses who protested were seen as "unscientific."

Whall (1989), incidentally, would assert that I am overstating the case. She has said that logical positivism did not have as much impact on nursing as is credited to it. To most of us, however, it seemed as if the narrow, logistic, borrowed wisdom was held as sacrosanct far too long—a function of our failure to move on with newer epistemologic theory.

As Suppe (1990) estimated, "Books in other disciplines which transmit the work of one discipline to readership within another discipline, are likely to be 10 years behind the cutting edge." (p. 1) Suppe, a philosopher, pointed out numerous theorists and ideas, no longer topical in their own fields, still holding sway in nursing. He cited Kuhn and Laudan as examples (p. 2), and, yes, logical positivism (p. 8).

The same case might be made presently for hermeneutics, already getting less attention in philosophy than in nursing. Or take the simpler notion of terms: *paradigm*—still heavily used in nursing—is being replaced elsewhere with the less pompous *construct*. Nursing's greatest vulnerability may be its tendency to rely heavily on other disciplines for its structure and methods.

Suppe (1990) also noted the tendency in nursing to equate scientific method with logical positivism, thereby claiming it as reductionistic and incompatible with holistic theory (p. 18). He noted two identity sets functioning in nursing:

Natural science = the scientific method = reductionistic = logical positivistic = quantitative
Human sciences = humanistic = antireductionistic = phenomenologic = qualitative (p. 19)

Suppe found both sets of equations untenable:

> Further, that positivistic account is built around two independent components, the so-called Received View on Theories (wherein theories are axiomatic deductive systems given a partial observational interpretation via correspondence rules), and the reductionistic thesis that all phenomena in principle can be explained in the most fundamental terms. . . . [T]hese are two independent theses about science (p. 19).
>
> The claim that logical positivism favors a quantitative approach is just false. For the Received View treats qualitative observational descriptions as most basic and fundamental; indeed the origins of positivism's Received View on Theories are in the problem how to erect quantitative theories on such a qualitative basis, and the Received View never did succeed in giving a fully satisfactory solution to the problem. Thus it is absolutely false that there is any intrinsic connection between logical positivism, the scientific method, and quantitative research techniques (p. 2).

Suppe separated phenomenology from qualitative methods, noting that descriptions for an entire sample population can be manipulated by quantitative statistical analyses. These historical attempts to make global, unnecessary connections between diverse concepts may account in part for the backlash against empirical research in nursing at present.

Gortner (1990) protested this unfair representation, saying about the literature on the so-called science of caring that

> in all but a few of these essays, science is cast against humanism and hermeneutics; the latter is seen as providing true meaning for all human endeavor including scientific work on humans and by humans (p. 102).

Her argument is not that hermeneutics has no place in nursing, but that its place is narrow, limited to certain nursing situations, and that those situations do not compose the totality of nursing. Her argument is that *understanding* (the goal of hermeneutics) does not replace *knowledge*—achieved by empirical research. As Gortner said,

> Human science activities cannot rest only with increased understanding; nor can that understanding be taken as the sole criterion for explanation as Benner has proposed. Human patterns and regularities and perhaps even "laws" characterize the human state and undergird the whole enterprise of society and human life. . . . [I]t is argued here that explication is a necessary requirement of nursing science as a clinical and human science, and that eventually such explanations will guide nursing action as therapy (p. 104).

Norbeck (1987) added, "When we make room for new perspectives, we must be careful not to throw away what is still useful from previous perspectives." (p. 29) She is not naive in her view of empiricism:

> One of the central challenges to the empiricist view, however, is that objective observation of human behavior, stripped from contextual meanings, is a violation of truth. . . . As an empiricist, I subscribe to the notion that there are observables "out there" that can be measured (p. 29).

The issue raised between supporters of empiricism versus advocates of phenomenology is an issue of ontology, of epistemology, and of research methods as well. To state the extreme cases, some researchers will forever be dissatisfied with a method that does not objectify and isolate variables. Such researchers will never grant that phenomenologic approaches can lead to knowledge. In contrast, many researchers with phenomenologic methods hold that much of what is true is lost in the very act of objectifying and isolating parts.

When one method, principle, or interpretation is taken as given and unassailable, it is possible, taking that stance, to criticize with impunity any theory based on another method, principle, or interpretation. Take, for example, the Nursing Theories Conference Group's (1980) criticism of Rogers's theory from the logistic perspective:

> Terms have not been sufficiently operationalized to provide for clear understanding. By operationalizing terms is meant the description of a set of physical procedures that must be carried out in order to assign to every case a value for the concept. For example, to operationalize the concept of width is to place a tool consisting of the units of inches or centimeters along the edge of the item to be measured and count the units.

Because of the lack of operational definitions, research done to support or verify the principles provides questionable results (p. 90).

Notice that the criticism of Rogers is essentially criticism that she is not using a logistic method. The eternal validity and correctness of the group's own method over Rogers' was never questioned, nor was it unusual in the nursing literature to find the same lecturing tone. Having escaped the stranglehold of the logistic empiricists, it is to be hoped that we will not see the pattern reversed, with those supporting phenomenologic methods equally zealous to support their methods at the cost of others.

SUMMARY

Despite its importance, this chapter decreases the amount of discussion of the relationships among theory, research, and knowledge from the last edition. The fact that such detailed information is not required any more is due to our growth as a profession. Today, this information is readily available in our nursing research literature, and that is the proper place for such discussions.

Still, it is impossible not to notice how research methods and theory preferences change as notions of reality change. Look at the changes, for example, accompanying the New Age paradigm. Or look at the way trends in methods affect content. As phenomenology evolved, developing specific methods of hermeneutics and critical social theory, these methods were accompanied by (I will not try to say which was cause, which effect) theories that focused on social consciousness.

Whatever theory a nurse employs, it is essential that she be able to discuss what world view it represents, as well as what research methods are appropriate given its content and context.

REFERENCES

Benner, P. (1985). Quality of life: A phenomenological perspective on explanation, prediction, and understanding in nursing science. *Advances in Nursing Science, 1,* 1–14.

Bergson, H. (1955). *An introduction to metaphysics.* New York: Bobbs-Merrill.

Cohen, M. Z. (1987). A historical overview of the phenomenologic movement. *Image, 1,* 31–34.

Dewey, J. (1938). *Logic: The theory of inquiry.* New York: Henry Holt.

Fawcett, J. (1978). The relationship between theory and research: A double helix. *Advances in Nursing Science, 1,* 49–62.

Gortner, S. (1990). Nursing values and science: Toward a science philosophy. *Image, 2,* 101–105.

Jacox, A. (1974). Theory construction in nursing—An overview. *Nursing Research, 1,* 4–13.

Kant, I. (1953). *Prolegomena to any future metaphysics* (P. G. Lucas, Trans.). Manchester, England: University of Manchester Press.

Kim, H. S. (1990, September). *Identifying alternative linkages among philosophy, theory, and method in nursing science.* Paper presented at the Symposia on Knowledge Development, University of Rhode Island College of Nursing, Kingston, RI.

Newman, M. A. (1992). Prevailing paradigms in nursing. *Nursing Outlook, 1,* 10–13.

Norbeck, J. S. (1987). In defense of empiricism. *Image, 1,* 28–30.

Nursing Theories Conference Group (Julia B. George, Chairperson). (1980). *Nursing theories: The base for professional nursing practice.* Englewood Cliffs, NJ: Prentice-Hall.

Paterson, J. G., & Zderad, L. T. (1976). *Humanistic nursing.* New York: Wiley.

Patterson, D. M. (1991, September). *Hermeneutics and the philosophy of praxis.* Paper presented at the Conference on Knowledge Development in Nursing, College of Nursing, University of Rhode Island College of Nursing, Kingston, RI.

Popper, K. R. (1953). The sociology of knowledge. In P. P. Wiener (Ed.), *Readings in philosophy of science* (pp. 357–366). New York: Charles Scribner's Sons.

Rabinow, P., & Sullivan, W. M. (1987). *Interpretive social science: A second look.* Berkeley: University of California Press.

Suppe, F. (1990, September). *Knowledge development in the context of shifting world views: The philosophy–theory linkage.* Paper presented at the Symposia on Knowledge Development, University of Rhode Island College of Nursing, Kingston, RI.

Webster, G., Jacox, A., & Baldwin, B. (1984). Nursing theory and the ghost of the received view. in J. C. McCloskey & H. Grace (Eds.), *Current issues in nursing* (pp. 26–35). Boston: Blackwell Scientific.

Whall, A. L. (1989). The influence of logical positivism on nursing practice. *Image, 4,* 243–245.

Appendix *A*

Analysis of an Extant Theory

This appendix analyzes a theory statement by Lydia Hall (1966), then director of the Loeb Center for Nursing and Rehabilitation at Montefiore Hospital and Medical Center, who would have been surprised to be termed a theorist. Yet Hall was a powerful one in that she had a unique concept of nursing, one that she was able to implement. One of the most important tests of a theory is its applicability in practice; hers met the test. Furthermore, it shows that nursing theory is not new; it has been with us longer than is often recognized.

Hall's (1966) theory appeared in *Continuity of Patient Care: The Role of* Nursing; the reader is invited to review that material firsthand. Theorists change their views over time, and different theory statements from the same author are likely to vary. Therefore, it is necessary to select a *particular* theory statement for analysis.

In a capsule, Hall made these important points before she presented her theory *per se*. One could label these underlying assumptions as follows:

- Professional services change to meet society's needs, and today's health problems focus on long-term illness.
- Medicine's role is *cure*, but this is inapplicable to long-term disease.
- For long-term illness, rehabilitation is required, shifting the patient from a passive to an active role.
- Because rehabilitation is an active role, learning is involved.

Barbara J. Stevens Barnum: NURSING THEORY:
ANALYSIS APPLICATION, EVALUATION, FOURTH EDITION.
© 1994, 1990, 1984, 1979 J.B. Lippincott.

- The nurse is *there* to do teaching; she has opportunity because of her ongoing presence for the ministering of personal care.

Hall covered this material in a single paragraph, but it gives the reflective reader a lot of information about the upcoming theory. The first point indicates that Hall's theory is delimited by time. If what professionals (and therefore nurses) do changes as societal needs change, then there is no absolute, eternal content of nursing. Hall may be classified with those theorists who say, *Nursing is what nurses do.* That position enables the content of nursing to shift over time.

This position also is action based, with the acts of the nurse assuming prominence over the specific knowledge content. Indeed, Hall confirmed this view when she addressed the nursing act of *teaching* rather than the *content* of what is to be taught.

Because what nurses do changes, Hall can give us a theory only for her time, that is, a time in which long-term illness was the dominant social health problem. Note that the article was published in 1966.

UNDERLYING ASSUMPTIONS

One of the analyst's first tasks is to recognize an author's underlying assumptions. Sometimes assumptions are not stated but can be inferred on the basis of other statements in the given work. Hall gives hers in the first paragraph.

Underlying assumptions are those basic premises accepted by the author as given, self-evident, and unquestioned. They describe that state of being out of which the nursing theory grows. Underlying assumptions, no matter where they appear in the written work, are the starting points of the author's reasoning.

It is important to identify underlying assumptions because they mark the boundary between internal and external criticism of a theory. For external criticism, the reader asks, Do the theorist's underlying assumptions ring true? Do they represent the real world, especially the real world of nursing? For internal criticism, the reader asks, Given the theorist's underlying assumptions, does her theory follow? Is it consistent with and logical in light of the underlying assumptions?

If a reader fails to differentiate between internal and external criticism, she may reject Hall's theory outright if she strongly objects to the premise that long-term care is the primary basis for nursing care. In rejecting the theory on this basis, a reader has failed to judge the theory on its own merits (i.e., whether it would be a good theory if that premise were true). A thorough criticism of a theory requires that attention be given to both internal and external criticism. It is possible for a reader to find a theory skillfully and consistently developed but arising out of premises that she cannot accept. Also, it is possible to find a theory having underlying assumptions with which a reader agrees, yet having a poorly developed argument. One might argue that Hall's position as director of a rehabilitation institution biases her perspective on the importance of long-term illness. This is an illustration of external criticism.

In Hall's five introductory points, she tends to differentiate roles and functions, for example, what medicine does, what the patient does, and what the nurse does. She discriminates between acts of persons or groups, a pattern of analysis often found in those authors who deal with the real nursing world. Having to act in the extant setting, Hall could hardly be expected to retreat into abstractions or global concepts of nursing.

Hall's fourth and fifth points present an interesting image of nursing. Rehabilitation is equated with teaching–learning, not with personal care. Personal care merely becomes an entry point, an excuse, so to speak, for the nurse's being there to teach.

In studying nursing theory, the reader learns to consider the implications and directions set in every sentence, reading slowly and thoughtfully, mining every paragraph for its significance. One cannot read for broad coverage in theory work.

HALL'S THEORY

Hall's theory says the following. A patient has three aspects of being: (1) body, (2) pathology and treatment, and (3) person. Medicine controls the aspect of pathology and treatment, and other professions, such as psychiatry, psychology, social work, and ministry, lay claim to the area of person. If nursing is to have an area of expertise, it must be the body. (Note Hall's need to differentiate professions by task and role.)

In examining the nurse's role as body expert, Hall says the intent of body care is comfort. But, she adds, not only does the body respond to such comfort, but so does the person. This enables the closeness of body care to become a medium for a learning experience in which the nurse becomes a nurturer. The nurse nurtures the patient toward better self-understanding and concomitant improved self-control. To use Hall's terms, through bodily care, the nurse helps the patient get to the core of his problems and sees him through the cure (medicine's domain). Hall's goal for the patient is self-knowledge and self-control as evidenced in his conscious choice of rewarding behavior. The nurse uses herself as a mirror in which the patient may learn to know himself and, in Hall's words, "change his behavior from sickness to wellness." Hall's theory still has great appeal for nurses. On the face of it, the theory has merit for at least two reasons: It defines a unique role for nurses (i.e., body experts) and it presents a positive view of patiency (i.e., a movement toward self-awareness).

Analysis of a theory, however, demands that one dig for a deeper insight into all its meaning and implications. The nurse must be able to point out flaws and inconsistencies. Lack of intelligent scrutiny allows poor theorists to flourish and does not help good ones to refine their work.

True, the critic has an unfair edge over the theorist; it is easier to find the flaws in works of others than to create one's own theory. Nursing owes a debt to those nurses willing to theorize. Criticisms are given in recognition of this fact.

Commonplaces

Only one set of commonplaces is applied to Hall's theory, starting with the nursing act. Of what does a *nursing act* consist for Hall? She differentiates between comforting (body care) and nurturing (teaching–learning). Although others may comfort, only the nurse nurtures. A nursing act is a teaching act. And what is taught? The subject matter is unusual, because teaching is normally perceived as transmission of cognitive knowledge. In Hall's theory, the subject is more properly an affective content, because the patient is taught self-knowledge and self-control. The nursing act for Hall is an act of education, in which the nurse teaches by serving as a mirror, reflecting self and self-awareness for the patient. Hall specifies that her nurses learn Rogerian counseling for this task.

Is this concept of a nursing act consistent throughout Hall's theory? Originally, she asserted that nurses were the body experts, but ultimately one finds that their focus is not body but person. Hall herself asserted that other professions *lay claim to* the person. If those claims were legitimate, how does the nurse justify leaving the area of body expertise to intervene in the area of person? (Surely self-awareness and self-knowledge have more to do with person than with body.)

Hall has let body care become a *means* to another *end*, that is, self-awareness and self-control. Body care becomes a mere medium that gets the nurse in the right position to act on the person. Ironically, this subjugation of body care to another end seems to denigrate nursing's area of expertise. The ultimate nursing act is that of inviting the patient to see himself and to choose (and thereby control) his own behavior.

Who or what fills the commonplace of *patient?* What differentiates him from nonpatients? Hall refers only to persons who happen to be admitted to health care facilities. Her image of a patient is of a hospitalized person, specifically one with a long-term illness.

What *characterizes* a patient, however, is his lack of full self-awareness and self-control. A problem arises from this unstated assumption. Is it always the case that an individual with a long-term illness loses control of his own fate? For Hall, it is assumed to be inevitable: a person with a long-term illness loses control—he becomes a patient.

The problem is one of differentiating patients from other people. Is the answer based on geography (hospitalized versus nonhospitalized persons) or is it based on the degree of self-awareness and self-control? One can imagine a deficiency in self-awareness in many persons walking the streets with healthy bodies. If Hall holds self-awareness as the criterion of patiency, she should concur that illness of body merely gives nurses the opportunity to assist a portion (a captive audience of sorts) of the whole class of patients, that is, those lacking self-awareness.

What is *health* for Hall? Health occurs when one masters self and consciously chooses one's own behaviors. Given this definition and given self-mastery as the goal of nursing, one can imagine a healthy paraplegic and an unhealthy star athlete. Note that Hall never equates self-mastery with mastery of the voluntary body; mastery relates to how one controls oneself given the environment and body in which one finds himself.

An existential goal is applied to patients having marked deficiencies of body structure and function, not unlike some of the more modern theories such as Watson's (1988) or Newman's (1986). One might argue that periods of body debilitation or pain bring about exactly the right circumstances for increasing self-awareness and introspection. Less charitably, a critic might say that Hall's nurses impose their values on the person when he is least able to resist their indoctrination due to physical debilitation.

What is the *relationship between nursing act and patient?* How do nurses relate to patients? Is the patient active or passive in the relationship? A tension exists here, because Hall's nurse *invites* the patient to achieve self-mastery. The patient is active in the sense that he can choose to master self or to reject the invitation (education). Nevertheless, the patient does not have ultimate control; the nurse *will* extend the invitation—whether or not it is desired. In this sense, she is manipulative and the patient is passive; he is a captive audience by virtue of his dependency on her for physical care.

Hall's theory is a nurse-based theory, focusing primarily on what the nurse does rather than on who the patient is or what he experiences. Nor is the focus on the nature of the interaction between patient and nurse. Ultimately, the nurse knows best here. She enforces—or attempts to enforce—her value of self-mastery on the patient.

How does the nursing act relate to health? The nursing act (nurturing, mirroring) is the catalyst for health. The nurse stimulates the patient to increase his own level of wellness. *How does the patient relate to health?* For Hall, health is behavior rather than a state of being. Good health is a goal toward which the patient can strive by increased self-awareness and increased self-control.

PROBLEMS OF ANALYSIS

Some readers may argue concerning this sort of analysis: It is not likely that the theorist gave her work this much attention when she wrote it. So it is unfair to seek deeper meanings in her work than those intended and hold her accountable for the specific and technical meanings of every word she may have used casually and informally.

The answer to this argument is three-fold. First, we can never know the author's intent, other than by reliance on the terms she selects and the meaning she gives them. Second, if a theorist is writing casually and without much thought, this sort of criticism will encourage her to tighten up her thinking. Third, and most important, seeking the deeper meaning and pertinent implications in theories is likely to have impact on the course of future nursing. To allow nursing practices to follow uncriticized fads and fashions is plainly hazardous.

Hall's theory illustrates another problem that often occurs. Many nurse leaders have been impressed by and have implemented Hall's concept of the nurse as body expert. Indeed, Hall elaborates on this concept, differentiating body care (comforting and nurturing) from medical care (cure) that involves the infliction of pain. Hall decries the misplaced desire of nurses to take on such medical tasks, becoming *potential painers* instead of *comforters* and *nurturers*.

Many nurses, influenced by the body expert/comforter aspect of Hall's theory, have adopted this isolated segment and claim to follow her theory. Clearly, this interpretation of Hall presents a case of *selective perception*. A casual reader of a theory often adopts the aspects of the theory that most interest her. These aspects may or may not be the most significant for the author.

Careful, unbiased reading of a theory is necessary to avoid selective perception, especially if the goal is to learn what the theorist says, not what the reader wishes had been said. The misinterpretation of Hall's theory is a case in point. For Hall, body care was simply a *means*; self-awareness and mastery was the *goal*. Many of her so-called followers selectively failed to hear this part of her theory. When one changes the *goal* of a theory, one has done radical surgery on the theorist's ideas.

This is not to say that a theory cannot be altered, but there must be recognition that surgery has been performed. Mere retention of Hall's vocabulary (e.g., painers, comforters, nurturers) is not retention of her theory. Always understand a theory *as given* before altering it.

REFERENCE

Hall, L. E. (1966). Another view of nursing care and quality. In K. M. Straub & K. S. Parker (Eds.), *Continuity of patient care: The role of nursing* (pp. 47–66). Washington, DC: Catholic University of America Press.

BIBLIOGRAPHY

Hall, L. E. (1955, February). *Quality of nursing care.* Paper presented at a meeting of the Department of Baccalaureate and Higher Degree Programs of the New Jersey League for Nursing, Newark, NJ.

Newman, M. A. (1986). *Health as expanding consciousness.* St. Louis, MO: C. V. Mosby.

Watson, J. (1988). Nursing: *Human science and human care: A theory of nursing.* New York: National League for Nursing.

Wiggins, L. R. (1980). Lydia Hall's place in the development of theory in nursing. *Image, 1,* 10–12.

Index

Twelve-step programs
  confrontation in, 224–225
  spirituality in, 117–118

U

Underlying assumptions
  of nursing practice, 33–35
  of nursing theory, 186–187, 284–285
Unitary vs. transformative paradigm, 270
Universal nursing theory, 8
Utility, of nursing theory, 4–5, 188, 190

V

Vaillot, Madeleine Clemence, 222
Validation, of theory, 273
Values, 7
  ethics and, 121
  in normative theory, 38–39
Venn diagram, 148, 183, 184
Vincent, K.G., 159
Vines, Susan W., 108, 109
Visintainer, Madelon A., 1
Visiting nurse, 41

W

Walker, Lorraine O., 148

Watson, Jean, 15, 22, 42, 77–80, 82, 89–91, 92, 95, 100, 103, 113, 119, 137, 196, 207, 208, 209, 210–211, 213, 215, 218, 287
Weber, R., 64, 65
Webster, Glen, 277
Weed charting, 161–162
Weiss, S., 64
Weissman, G., 236
Wellness, 42
Welt, S.R., 216
Werley, H.H., 153
Whall, Ann L., 148, 205, 277
White, J.A., 108
Wiedenbach, E., 75–76
Wilber, K., 79, 204
Wolf, Zane Robinson, 72–73
Wood, Dolores Jean, 88, 95, 155
Work motifs, 244

Z

Zablow, Robin J., 123
Zahourek, Rothlyn, 108
Zderad, Loretta T., 135, 218, 223, 225, 275
Zetterlund, Joan, 133
Ziman, John, 27